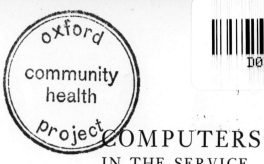
COMPUTERS
IN THE SERVICE
OF MEDICINE

VOLUME I

Essays on current research
and applications

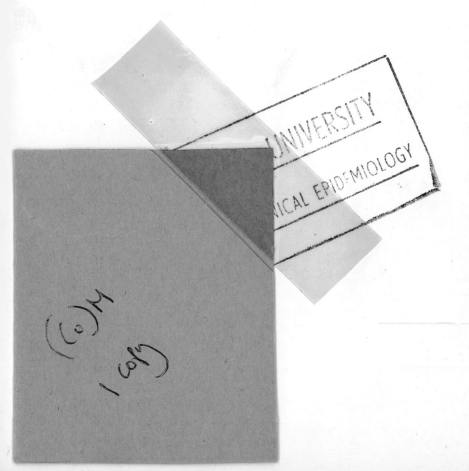

COMPUTERS
IN THE SERVICE
OF MEDICINE

VOLUME I

Essays on current research and applications

EDITED BY GORDON McLACHLAN
AND RICHARD A. SHEGOG

Published for the Nuffield Provincial Hospitals Trust
by the Oxford University Press 1969
London New York Toronto

Oxford University Press, Ely House, London W1

GLASGOW NEW YORK TORONTO MELBOURNE WELLINGTON
CAPE TOWN SALISBURY IBADAN NAIROBI LUSAKA ADDIS ABABA
BOMBAY CALCUTTA MADRAS KARACHI LAHORE DACCA
KUALA LUMPUR HONG KONG TOKYO

First printed 1968, reprinted 1969

Cover design by Edward Bawden C.B.E., R.A.
Designed by Bernard Crossland
Printed in Great Britain by Alden & Mowbray Ltd
at the Alden Press, Oxford

Bound by Kemp Hall Bindery, Oxford

Preface

by BRIAN H. FLOWERS, F.R.S.
Chairman of the Science Research Council
Chairman Computer Board for Universities and Research Councils

It is now commonplace that computers are likely to affect us, directly or otherwise, in many aspects of our lives. They have become indispensable in almost all branches of science and technology whether research, development or production. They are becoming of increasing importance in quantitative planning, in economics and transport for example, and in the evaluation of strategy whether military or civil. As the technology for computing develops—and it has developed at a phenomenal rate in the past few years—it is becoming possible to talk in sensible terms of the immense problems of data storage and information retrieval. The essential requirements here, of course, are vast amounts of quick access memory, and the facility to extract and add to it simultaneously from many places at any time. Fast arithmetic was the first stage of the computer revolution; multi-access is the second.

The articles which follow this brief introduction tell the story of the gradual invasion of computers into medicine. I am not competent to judge in any detail the nature of the medical need nor to comment specifically upon the way that need is being met. However, many of the problems discussed here, both of hardware and of software, are not unique to medicine and it therefore seems important that they should not be seen in isolation. No science could be more interdisciplinary than the application of computers and much may be gained from cross-fertilization between applications in different fields. Teaching hospitals in universities which are already computer conscious in a variety of ways can be expected to play an important part in pioneering medical computing, and it is therefore no surprise that several of these articles originate from the teaching hospitals. It is easy to be ambitious, and common enough to be over-ambitious, in planning a computer facility: only too often the limitation proves to be a human one, shortage of staff or failure sufficiently to define the task. It is equally easy, though perhaps less common nowadays, to be under-ambitious through lack of knowledge of what computers can do in a new context or simply by being wedded to the well-tried methods of the past. It may well be necessary to change established procedures far down the line before the computer can be seen to be worthwhile. Interaction with other disciplines provides a broader background of experience against which detailed schemes can be evaluated.

Someone has said recently that after several years of vigorous growth computing is now approaching its infancy. Certainly it is still a highly experimental discipline, and one in which a flexible approach is essential. Too much standardization of equipment or procedures at the present stage could be wasteful in the longer term. Now that it is becoming possible to link small machines to large ones the teaching hospitals again have an advantage: some of them already have access to large university machines, and it may prove possible to limit their own capital equipment to the link and the satellite at least until the nature of the problem is better understood.

Computers of a former generation were unsophisticated devices difficult to programme. Increasingly sophisticated hardware and software have made the user's job much easier: for simple jobs such as bank entries and flight-reservations he no longer has to be an expert programmer. I suspect that the medical needs are much more difficult to meet, especially since the failure rate must be extremely low. In these circumstances it may be some time before a satisfactory standard system is available at a reasonable price. In the meantime the medical user must be prepared to be sophisticated, both in his use of equipment and in his evaluation of the current needs.

The techniques of computing have been developed so far largely in response to the needs of physical scientists, engineers, and accountants. Physicists, mathematicians, engineers and accountants are plentiful in the computer industry: many of them have been users in their time. Doctors in the computer industry are rare except as medical officers. Medical computing would come more quickly into its own if some doctors could be persuaded to join the industry. I suspect that industry would welcome them.

Contents

I

Introducing a computer to a hospital

Experiences of the experiment
at Birmingham

E. G. KNOX

Managing a computer service

E. G. Knox, M.D., M.R.C.P.

Senior Lecturer in Social Medicine
University of Birmingham

Introducing a computer to a hospital

Experiences of the experiment at Birmingham

In December 1966, after three years of study and preparation, a computer system was installed in the Medical School at Birmingham University to serve the joint needs of the United Birmingham Hospitals and the Faculty of Medicine. It was specified in the main to meet data-processing needs rather than large-scale calculations and the central equipment, an IBM 1440, is neither a large nor very fast machine. It has only a 16K character store—the largest available for this model—but it possesses a good range of input/output devices including a card reader/punch, a paper tape reader, two magnetic tape decks, two magnetic disc drives with interchangeable disc packs, and a line printer.

The purpose of this paper is to describe the process of its introduction rather than the purposes to which it is being put, and to describe the range of problems encountered in the process.

Initial justification

The initial justification for the joint project was that both the Hospital Group and the Medical School needed large-scale data-processing facilities unavailable elsewhere, and that the experience of their staffs in computing and data-processing methods was adequate for its success.

The background was that (*a*) the Birmingham University computer could not at that time meet these needs (no card reader, no line printer, no direct access magnetic storage device, inadequate ancillary equipment, no Cobol or Fortran compilers); (*b*) there was already a well-developed automatic document preparation facility using punch cards, in the Department of Biochemistry, where auto-analyser techniques had been used for some time; (*c*) there was considerable research usage and experience of automatic data-processing methods in several of the university departments, particularly Anatomy, Experimental Pathology, and Social Medicine; (*d*) several departments had experience of automatic digitisation of analogue data, particularly Medicine, Neurocommunications, and Neuropharmacology; (*e*) a Hospital Management Services Unit had been studying patterns of data flow and new methods of managerial control; these depended upon the automatic acquisition and manipulation of information.

The purposes of the project were listed under five headings:

Education and training in computer methods.
Research.
The development of computer methods in patient care and record keeping.
The development of automated laboratory methods.
The development and integration of improved managerial/ financial techniques.

The sequence of events

The first written proposals were produced for the project in August 1964. The Board of the Faculty of Medicine and the Board of Governors of the Teaching Hospitals approved the proposals and established a Computing Facilities Steering Committee representing the two authorities. It was agreed that the project should be a joint one, but that the administrative responsibility for the computer should be accepted by the University through the Department of Social Medicine. More detailed studies of requirements were then carried out and in April 1965 the Steering Committee invited four computer firms to make their own assessments of needs, and to make proposals. By November their proposals had been received and studied, and a decision on equipment made. This decision was influenced considerably by the practical considerations of immediate availability and the probable scale of available finance. The main need was seen to be for a modest machine upon which experience could be built from an early date, rather than a larger one which could not be implemented or justified for some time.

In March 1966 definitive proposals were put to the Nuffield Provincial Hospitals Trust and accepted. A grant of £60 000 was made to cover the installation and hire of main equipment, to employ the staff to run it, and to contribute towards alterations of premises. It was expected that the grant would be sufficient for two years' work.

There still remained the task of obtaining finance from other sources for ancillary equipment, furnishings, expendables, and additional personnel, but the main grant made it possible to go ahead with ordering equipment, modifying premises, and advertising for staff. The senior staff were appointed in July, the computer room prepared by November and junior staff appointed; the computer, together with a first set of ancillary equipment, was delivered before the end of 1966.

CRITICAL PATHS

This presentation of the sequence of events affords little indication of the complexity of the processes required to bring them about. It can be seen that there were three main 'streams of acquisition' relating to equipment, staff, and premises. Each required detailed planning on its own account and the timings and contingencies of each stream interacted with the management of the other two. In addition several lines of systems design were necessary and they in turn reacted with each other and with each of the main acquisitive processes.

It is possible to present this pattern as a 'network analysis', or 'critical path analysis' of decisions and actions, but this technique was not in fact used as a planning device. The environment of the project was not one in which absolute control of all stages and decisions could be allotted to a small executive group to permit detailed advance planning of this type, and all of the main executive streams were at times so tentative and mutually dependent that it was not possible to delineate all the ways in which the project might go.

As a retrospective description of what actually happened a network analysis would be quite fraudulent. One discrepancy between
it and the actual operation is that the network has a clearly defined
beginning and end, whereas the actual process of introducing the
computer was less definite, with a rather vague beginning, and no
end yet in sight. Furthermore the exact definition of the reasons for
taking particular steps often seemed to crystallize after they had
occurred, rather than before. The network fails to express this, and
the feeling that particular points had been passed before; the growth
of the project seemed often to follow a circular or spiral, rather than
a linear pattern.

The imagery of an executive process has some importance for its
acceptability and success and too detailed and rigid a plan might
have failed to cater for growth potential, and for the necessary
flexibility of development.

With these reservations it may be safe, as a textual convenience,
to pursue separately the three main 'streams of acquisition' and to
describe the problems involved.

Equipment

Computing equipment comes in large steps. The pressures which
this fact imposed upon the Birmingham project are likely to apply to
similar enterprises, and although the first step is the largest, we have
found that these pressures apply also to subsequent upgradings of
equipment. These pressures are (*a*) to step up the level of anticipated
initial usage before the equipment arrives, (*b*) to delay delivery while
this is done, and (*c*) to reduce the scale of equipment towards the
requirements of those applications which are specifically foreseen.

Raising the level of initial usage. A satisfactory solution here
depends upon the existence of previously defined proposals for
hospital data analysis and presentation, partly upon existing and
outstanding research problems, but largely upon progress in designing new systems and new research projects. Unfortunately it was
and is no more practical to invest in systems designs requiring a
computer, without the assurance that a computer will be obtained,
than it is to invest in equipment without being assured of its use,

and at the stage of negotiating their joint promotion the matter must hinge largely upon the experience and skills of persons already on the staff.

An early attempt was made to assess existing research requirements by means of questionnaire studies supplemented by informal talks, and a list of over thirty major research projects was prepared. It was necessarily somewhat contrived in that the respondents could not be told what configuration might be supplied nor when it might arrive. In the event several of the jobs were completed on other equipment, some aborted altogether, and others could not be suitably developed on the equipment which was eventually obtained. Other projects developed under the more realistic stimulus of the actual equipment when it did arrive and the count of current research projects is about that envisaged, although few of the items coincide specifically.

Similar uncertainties occurred in the processing of hospital service data. The payroll was a greater problem than anticipated and was delayed, while the registration system progressed with remarkable speed and was operational within five months. Biochemical quality control progressed very rapidly, but the file-handling system was more complex than was thought. The transfer of radiotherapy dosage calculations from other equipment involved considerable re-programming. Bed-state control data evolved rapidly once the registration system worked, but the linkage of management and finance data has proved to be a very large problem indeed.

Advance systems designs are clearly desirable when possible, before the computer arrives, but our experience has been that the tractability of different data-handling systems cannot confidently be predicted, nor can accurate estimates be made of the man-years of work necessary; the availability of systems staff must also be counted among the uncertainties. The unsatisfactory truth of the matter is that the early decisions had to be made upon essentially intuitive grounds and that the main basis had to be the number and quality of workers already using computers.

It is clear that a certain amount of experience was necessary even to make proposals for a computer system. When the Birmingham system was ordered about ten people in the hospital and in the

Faculty of Medicine had programming experience and their combined knowledge covered the use of six or seven different computers and as many programming languages and variations. Their joint experience included the use of cards and paper tape both for programming and for data input, the use of magnetic tape and of random access filing devices, and experience (from a users' point of view) of facilities at half a dozen different university and commercial centres. Three or four had fairly extensive experience going back for some years and were in a position to run programming courses and assist colleagues in programming problems. In addition to those with computer experience there was a larger number with experience of handling punch-card equipment, and in one department a considerable experience of automatic report writing in association with extensive use of automated laboratory equipment. Three departments had experience of conversion of the output of automatic laboratory equipment into digital form.

It is difficult to specify what is a proper level of development to be expected in a centre before it installs a computing facility of its own and this account is presented as a factual statement of a level which has proved reasonably satisfactory at Birmingham with a small computer, rather than as a statement of the optimum or minimum.

Delivery delays. There were problems in timing the arrival of main equipment, ancillary equipment, and staff. These problems too are likely to be general. It was necessary first to sign contracts so that delivery schedules could be initiated with a provisional view to the arrival of the computer about six months later. At that distance it was not possible to be sure that the other streams of acquisition and systems design could be completed in time, but it was not necessary or possible to decide on a definite delivery date at this stage. More acute problems arose when definite delivery options were offered for a major part of the equipment at a range of eight to twelve weeks.

At this stage there seemed little hope of making full use of the facility if it arrived on time, but the view was taken that delay might not have the intended effect of improving the state of preparation.

Enthusiastic workers might lose their enthusiasm—particularly as this was not the first of the delays—and there was the danger not only that less work would be done but that momentum would be lost. There were in hand one or two large simple jobs—it was decided to print the Hospital Diagnostic Index for the last ten years—and this provided some insurance. In addition, the normal law of progress with computing facilities is that the demand doubles annually; a reasonable minimum period for keeping a computer is something over two years so that even when a machine is half used when it first arrives, its over-all disabilities during its lifetime are that it is not big enough and that it arrived too late.

In practice there were further imposed delays, and when the machine arrived there was sufficient work to keep it fully occupied almost from the beginning.

It is usual practice among computer suppliers to offer free time on a bureau machine—in the case of the 1440, a total of twenty hours. Other users may find this more useful than we did, but the nearest bureau 1440 was a hundred miles away, it did not have the same configuration as the scheduled machine, and whatever the frustrations a computer may offer in its early days when actually on site, they are nothing compared with the problems it can offer on such a basis. With the relatively clear-cut problems of transferring a well-defined system, such as the radiotherapy dosage programmes previously operational on another machine, this time was useful, but not for the wider range of ill-defined systems to be developed.

This service could not provide an adequate substitute for on-site equipment and we have never regretted pressing for early delivery.

Reducing the scale of equipment. How large a computer to obtain was a difficult question dependent both upon the scale of probable finance and upon the degree of definition achieved with respect to the jobs to be tackled. These matters have already been examined. However, another factor bearing upon this was the question of buying or hiring. Clearly, a flexible means of disposing of equipment, or altering its configuration, permits a start to be made at a stage of development where long-term commitments to a particular machine or size of machine could not be contemplated. Some firms offer a form of hire purchase, which may be helpful if capital funds are short, but we regarded this as equivalent to purchase since it did not provide the flexibility of a hire agreement.

These problems can now be avoided to some extent in the new generation of computers but it is not always true that a machine can be enlarged smoothly by adding modules. And it is not possible, if the equipment has been purchased, readily to change the nature of the configuration—say by replacing magnetic tape with interchangeable discs, or disposing of discs and replacing by magnetic card file.

The essence of the project was that it was an experiment in a working context, and one of its objectives was to find the best configuration; the view was taken that a flexible hiring system had more to offer towards this end than purchase.

The cost of the machine was not unfavourable on a hire—as opposed to purchase—agreement. In practice the equipment is charged for at about 40 per cent of its normal rate since IBM gave a 60 per cent 'academic contribution' towards the experimental purposes to which it is largely put. However, this would have applied equally to a purchase agreement so did not unduly influence the choice. The annual cost is about one quarter of the purchase price but this includes maintenance which on a purchased machine could be a heavy additional financial item. Indeed, in situations where a machine will meet requirements for less than four years, and where its resale value is likely to be small, hiring may seem to be remarkably economic. We have found only one disadvantage. A hire agreement will not usually specify a new machine and the user may obtain one which has already been heavily used; in the present instance, the machine was no longer in production, so this was inevitable. It is true that a hired machine is 'reconditioned'—and that the central processor may be thought of as having an almost indefinite life—but a good deal of trouble might yet be anticipated from card readers, card punches, disc drives, tape-decks, paper tape readers, printers, etc. Most 'down time' has been from these units and it has been more than that expected from a new machine.

The 1440 was expected to meet most needs for about two years and possibly less, but the demand for computing developed more rapidly than anticipated. Within two weeks of its installation it was working a full shift and after six months approximately sixty hours per week.

This experience suggests that prior estimates of computer capacity required (staff as well as premises) should have been multiplied by some arbitrary factor between two and four.

This seems to be one of the facts of life and doubtless is well known to computer salesmen. In contrast with other walks of life, where a salesman tries to sell more than is needed, he tries here to sell less. He knows that the lesser estimates will be accepted more readily and that he will in any case be approached for more equipment before very long.

Staff

For most of the time the staff has comprised a manager, a senior systems analyst, a senior programmer and a programmer, a computer operator, and two punch operators. There was an additional programmer for part of the time and some secretarial assistance has been borrowed from one of the university departments. In addition a good deal of card punching has been done in departments which were already equipped to do it.

The chief weakness of this staffing structure is at machine-room level. Holidays, weekends, sickness, backlogs, resignations at operator/programmer level mean that senior staff have to spend too much of their time keeping the system running. There should be in addition a computer room supervisor, an additional operator, two extra programmers, and at least one other systems analyst. The number of punch operators required depends upon the degree of centralization, but this too would be a more efficient process if there were three more.

The competition for staff was severe. Starting salaries for managers and senior systems analysts are between £1900 and £2200, senior programmers £1100–1900, programmers, computer room supervisors, and systems analysts £900–1400, operators £600-800 and punch operators £400-600. The payroll for the staff considered necessary for optimum running of the unit, together with their Social Security and Superannuation contributions, would be between £16 000 and £17 000 per annum initially, plus increments and rises.

These requirements were underestimated at the planning stage and current annual expenditure is about £10 000.

Another problem of staff acquisition was in appointment grades. Computing is a new profession and existing staff gradings both in university and hospital are imperfectly adapted. For example the senior technician and technician grades in the hospital and university have age-linked maximum salaries and may be dependent upon technical qualifications not strictly relevant to computing, and university academic grades usually depend upon holding a degree. This was particularly difficult at the senior programmer level where the applicants generally possessed *either* a degree *or* adequate practical experience, but not both. The manager and senior systems analyst have been employed on university administrative grades and programmers and operators on university programmer and operator grades. This is proving satisfactory so long as the University continues to act as the administrative agent for the project but there will be considerable problems in attracting and holding sufficient staff of sufficient quality on existing non-medical grades within the Health Service.

Advertising and staff training were the two remaining problems of the 'staff acquisition stream'. They were not so much problems as unexpectedly large expenses. The senior positions required large-panel advertisements in the national daily and Sunday newspapers on more than one occasion. Training courses were also expensive involving course fees plus a month's residence in London and weekend travelling. Even highly qualified staff may not have experience of the particular equipment installed and junior staff must often be accepted as trainees, and a succession of training and retraining operations may be necessary.

Premises

It was estimated that the minimum practicable space for the installation in purpose designed premises would be about 2000 sq. ft. and that in existing premises, if the room sizes were not ideal this might need to be more. The space available for the computer itself, a lecture theatre, had a floor space of 600 sq. ft. and this has proved adequate for the 1440, together with some cabinets and a table or two. Because of the expense of conversion, and the desirability of avoiding a change of premises at some future date with transfer to larger equipment, a larger room would have been better, say 800 sq. ft.

The necessary modifications included false flooring and air conditioning with temperature and humidity control. The first humidifier was of the atomizer type and spread a fine white dust of lime from the water; it had to be replaced by an evaporation-type humidifier. Electrical rewiring was necessary and smoke and fire detectors were installed. Double glazing and acoustic ceiling were not fitted on grounds of expense and time. An automatic carbon dioxide extinguishing system was suggested but not fitted; there seemed to be some danger of extinguishing the staff.

The cost of modifying this room in time, in an adequate but less than ideal manner, was about £5000. For new premises the estimated building cost is about £12. 10s. 0d. per square foot, that is £7500 altogether.

Existing premises offered better economies where the necessary modifications were less extensive. Two rooms were obtained adjacent to the computer room and expenses here were measured in hundreds rather than in thousands of pounds. The first is an ancillaries room containing a counter-sorter, four card punches, two verifiers, two paper tape preparation machines and a punch-card duplicator with mark-sense attachments. The punch operators work here but it is also a public room where users or their technicians can prepare data and conduct some off-line processing. It is a noisy and crowded room of 300 sq. ft. serving also as a through room to the computer, and part of the floor area is taken up with a ramp to the false floor level of the computer room. Two rooms of this size would have been more suitable for this purpose.

The second room is a 'quiet' room of 250 sq. ft. used for reference to manuals, pondering over programmes, discussion over programming problems between users and professional programmers, and for the professional programmers to work in. This contains standard furnishings.

The computer unit is very much like a factory and the staff each have several work places. In addition to the computer room and its adjacent suite they must have somewhere which is neither noisy nor public where they can work on their own and where they can conduct interviews and consultations without disturbing each other unreasonably. There must also be a fair amount of storage space. Some of it can be in the computer room and some in the adjacent rooms but bulky supplies of cards, printer stationery, and special stationery—some of it, duplicating paper, requiring dry and temperature-controlled dark storage—requires some additional space. The rooms for these purposes need not necessarily be close to the computer and the floor area required depends to some extent upon the existing layout of available rooms but it is unlikely that these functions can be met in less than 600 sq. ft. of space and 800–1200 sq. ft. is probably more realistic, bringing the total for the unit to between 2000 and 2400 sq. ft. The difficulties of providing this amount of space from existing premises were always appreciated, and in fact it has not proved possible to supply all that was wanted. A difficult compromise in terms of space was the necessary price for an early start but for subsequent stages of the project new buildings will be necessary. With a larger computer the need for seminar/conference facilities, larger staff and increased centralization of data-preparation we estimate that 6000–9000 sq. ft. of space will be required.

OPERATIONS

In some senses a computer is a hospital service, like the central heating or a typing pool. It can perform many simple but tedious clerical tasks with speed, accuracy, and legibility. Many such tasks are simple in concept, often similar to well-understood work in other contexts than the hospital, and for their establishment as computer processes well within the competence of 'organization and methods' staff, aided by experienced systems analysts and programmers.

In other senses the computer is a tool to be used by the different professional groups within the hospital and medical school; administrators, doctors, nurses, technicians, pharmacists, physicists, and so on. Its applications are extensions and rationalizations of particular professional activities in whose development some of them must participate, and the resulting operations will in any case impinge upon the work of those who do not take part in active development. Therefore, although the adequacy and proper deployment of professional computing staff is essential to the development of computing methods in a hospital, much also depends upon the particular interests and experience of the main users and the best hope of progress is in reinforcing and supporting their work. Where they cannot be helped, they should at least not be hindered. Since it is not possible to advance uniformly over the whole field of possible operations, the aim should be for patchy success and the correct strategy is to reinforce achievement.

It is sometimes held that the development of computing in hospitals should be almost entirely a matter for professional computing staff; such considerable faith is placed in the abilities of trained systems analysts that systems designs are seen largely to be outside the competence of the doctors, nurses and others affected. The difference in approaches is important because the corollaries are different patterns of progress.

The first approach demands active participation of medical administrative and other hospital staff, a modest computing staff and several stages of equipment and re-equipment, beginning with a relatively small machine at an early stage. The second approach demands a large systems staff, a substantial period of analysis, the design of a total information flow pattern before equipment is specified, and a relatively late delivery of a large machine.

The Birmingham project uses the first approach and developments are conceived as parts of a planetary system, working towards rather than from a 'total information system', and permissive in the sense that departments can proceed at their own speed without offence to or hindrance from other departments, according to their abilities, needs, enthusiasms, and the tractability of their problems.

At the same time it has been recognized that developments in one area of work may very well affect progress in another and it has been necessary so to arrange matters that an unfortunate choice of file design, or of patient-identification data, or of programming language, does not later lead to incompatibility between systems which ideally should link, or compromise the transferability of a system to a later computer or to an application elsewhere. In addition the need for priority decisions between projects competing for limited machine time and limited staff resources has been anticipated. Such discretionary activities are needed not only as a negative process, but in order to fill any important gaps in the effort which might prejudice long-term success (for example, the need for common analogue–digital conversion techniques, interdepartmental filing compatibilities, reallocation of responsibilities following resignations, compatible stationery designs, etc.).

In such policy matters the problem has usually been definable as a zone or area of work, rather than one of the highly localized points at which progress is occurring at any one time. The problem then is how to control, balance, and encourage work in such zones without discouraging or inhibiting work at points within them. Particularly it is necessary to avoid a parcelling out of work in such a way as to inhibit enterprise in individuals with new ideas, either because they are made to feel that they are poaching on someone else's territory, or because they believe that the field is being developed so comprehensively that their efforts are not necessary.

We have tried to develop, and are still developing, an administrative system to meet these needs. It is not an easy task. Computers evoke emotions which other equipment does not, and they bring together people from different disciplines whose terminologies can raise difficulties of communication. Misunderstandings have stemmed from different meanings being attached to the terms 'systems analysis', 'hospital information system', 'registration file'—or because we failed for a time to specify the difference between 'patient identification' and 'record identification'. The 'who-does-what' problems arising from such misunderstandings sound trivial, and after they have been cleared up it is even embarrassing to mention them, but their diagnosis and resolution can be as difficult as any programming problem.

In addition a joint project between university and hospital raises problems of 'who-works-for-whom'. University staff without hospital appointments are drawn into service problems and invest large amounts of work and time without security of recognition for themselves or their departments. Hospital staff may feel that their work is in danger of being published as part of a university research project. None of this matters in the early enthusiastic days, but as investment mounts from weeks to years of staff time, and the computer project becomes for many a major commitment, a definitive method of resolving (and if possible preventing) such difficulties becomes a necessity. We have tried to meet the various problems of co-ordination, control, encouragement, and support, and to provide accountability for the project as a whole, through the following administrative organization.

1. **A Medical Centre Computing Committee** represents the hospital and the university with representatives both from the Faculty of Medicine and from the University Computing Committee. It makes major policy decisions upon the basis of information and advice from its parent bodies and from its Executive Committee (see below). It meets about once in six months.

2. **A Computer Executive Committee** is responsible to the main Committee and is appointed by it. It is not intended to be representative but its members are in close contact with all the main users. It meets once per month and its function is the immediate direction and control of the project. It was concerned in the specification and ordering of the equipment, the negotiations for funds, the appointment of staff, and the allocation and preparation of the available premises. It is concerned with specifying the next machine, the future staff structure, the premises required, and the pattern of work to be undertaken. It reviews usage of machine and staff time, adjudicates upon major applications for facilities, classifies and overlooks current usage, receives reports upon specific projects and is responsible for assessing and reporting upon their various successes and failures.

3. **The manager** is responsible for providing a day-to-day computing service, and the scheduling of operations, for first-hand relationships with suppliers of equipment and expendables, for appointment of junior staff and the allocation of their work and working time, and

for the security of the premises and equipment. He allocates expenditures to the various accounts. He is a member of the Executive Committee.

The manager has authority to approve projects which he judges to be of a minor nature but he is protected from undue pressure in that he can refer to the Executive Committee for a decision, projects likely to require a large proportion of facilities. Requests for special peripherals or ancillaries and special stationery are also dealt with in this way.

The senior systems analyst is his deputy.

4. **Users.** Individual projects are registered by agreement with the manager and/or Executive Committee and an initial declaration is made of the objectives and the anticipated use of machine facilities and requirements for central staff assistance. At a later stage, either on termination of the project as a whole or at the end of the stage of intensive development, a report is provided by the user. Meanwhile his actual use of facilities is logged.

Large and complex jobs, particularly those dependent upon co-operative efforts, have sometimes been defined as working-party projects and a working group with a chairman, rather than an individual user or department, is registered as responsible for the work. Some were established well before the computer arrived. At present there are six such groups, three engaged on various parts of the development of the patient records, one concerned with administration and finance, and two with central services (particularly software developments, sub-routine libraries, library (book) services, and Fortran usage).

FUTURE DEVELOPMENTS

Real achievements must be measured in terms of the research applications of the computer, and the development of data systems within the Hospital, rather than the administrative and organizational concepts presented in this paper, but their description is not within present purposes. This excuse at least is needed if we try to plot the future of the project without saying what has so far been achieved. Nevertheless this does in a sense represent the reality of the situation for we have found, and expect that others will find, that we were compelled to devise future plans before present ones had matured. The time-scales of delivery of equipment, the preparation of premises, and the development of information systems are such that it is necessary to plan the extension of an establishment and the replacement of equipment almost on the day that it arrives.

It is no bad thing that systems should develop in the shadow of their own obsolescence and that the designers of data-handling methods in the hospital should always have one eye on the possible shapes of ideas and equipment two or three years hence, but it makes life no easier for them. Constant efforts to improve the generalization of file handling and programme logic, to avoid methodological blind alleys in the structure of information collected, to avoid committal to a particular range of central or peripheral equipment, and to develop methods which will have general rather than local application, all multiply the programming effort required, reduce the machine-time efficiencies of programmes and add to the complexity of the liaison and compatibility problems between different departments.

The present is always competing with the future, the need for immediate and demonstrable returns pressing upon the need for maintaining a clear path ahead.

However, after a year of existence, nine months of computer operation, and the successful establishment of several systems associated with the hospital registration procedure, in the preparation of laboratory results, in the payroll system, in radiation dose calculations, and the replacement of a number of clerical tasks associated with the book-keeping of ward occupancy, the daily bulletin of patient states, the ambulance discharge list, etc., we are exploring the different ways of handling and servicing an integrated patient-record system.

Already our present equipment and staffing limit these developments. Using on the one hand the currency of our present usage of machine time and programming and systems efforts, and on the other hand the disparity between what we have so far achieved and that which we hope to achieve, it is already clear that the size of the establishment necessary for a hospital group is far larger than we ourselves envisaged. Moreover, we do not believe that this arithmetic has been faced squarely by many who have entered or hoped to enter this field. Amid the general talk of what computers can do in hospitals and other health services, there has been little realization of the power of the computer or the extent of the systems and programming work needed to achieve the aims, nor of the proportion of Health Service expenditure which would have to be allocated for these purposes.

The present Birmingham establishment spends the equivalent of 1 per cent of the budget of the United Birmingham Hospitals. However it is extremely difficult to present a realistic costing since part of the usage is for academic purposes while the equipment has been obtained at a large discount. Moreover, the limitations of the equipment and the absence of telecommunications prevented the computing service from being extended to the whole of the hospital group. Current expenditures might more properly be expressed in relation to those of the particular hospitals serviced. However, despite these costing problems, expenditures of the order quoted can almost certainly be expected to provide comparable increases in hospital efficiency, and in general terms are justified.

For the future, however, the problem of appraisal in terms of value for money is very difficult. An integrated information system on a hospital group basis (say 3000 beds altogether), using multiple immediate access terminals, might require expenditure on staff and equipment equivalent annually to 4 per cent of the budget. This should cover development as well as running costs and some retrenchment might eventually be possible, but once a computer system is installed new uses tend to be found, and the centres engaged in such development require allocations which, in the local context of running a hospital, are very large sums indeed. Such expenditures demand more exact estimates of value than those on a '1-per-cent level', and at the same time it can be asserted that, while 1-per-cent level improvements of efficiency might be very difficult to demonstrate, the 4 per cent plus improvements necessary to justify the larger equipments, should be more readily demonstrable.

Unfortunately the frame of reference within which value must be assessed does not coincide with that within which the expenditure is incurred and administered. The dislocation of these frames of reference occurs both in time and in space. First, the benefits can accrue only some time after the major part of the investment, and although projections can be made, only measured effects can be credible in the long run. Second, an increased efficiency of use of hospital resources might make the hospital more expensive to operate on a day basis, since more patients might be treated and the rate of expenditure upon patients concentrated into fewer days. It is true that there may be some relief of pressure in other parts of the Health Service and that some benefits might be demonstrable if assessments could be made from a wider point of view than the hospital board-room, but this still may not be evident in financial terms. The gearing of a service to deal more effectively with demands which it could not otherwise meet, is bound to make it more expensive to run.

In the end it seems inevitable that appraisals of value for money, from computers in hospitals and health services, will be in qualitative terms. If prior justifications are required in terms of financial saving, then, no doubt, projected estimates can be prepared, but the actual measurement of financial benefits will prove difficult or impossible except at selected points. More usually the benefits will be expressed in terms of quality, speed, and accuracy, and the provision of services would not otherwise have been possible—such as daily quality control of biochemical laboratory data, efficient waiting-list management, reduced days in hospital, prompt and error-free information to general practitioners that their patients have been discharged.

It will be more practical, profitable, and appropriate to the context, to try to declare what services have been obtained for the money spent, than to hope to demonstrate money saved. Ultimate decisions upon the scale of application of computers in health services will depend not upon their profitability, but upon their value, and upon competing claims made in similar terms by alternative proposals for investment.

2

Electronic processing of hospital records

K.W.CROSS
J.DROAR
J.L.ROBERTS

*Developing a new
communications system*

K. W. Cross, B.Sc., Ph.D.

Senior Lecturer, Department of Social Medicine
University of Birmingham
and Head of Hospital Statistics Department
United Birmingham Hospitals

J. Droar

Head of Management Services Unit
United Birmingham Hospitals

J. L. Roberts, B.Soc.Sc., A.H.A.

Senior Research Associate
Department of Social Medicine
University of Birmingham
and Statistician
United Birmingham Hospitals

Electronic processing of hospital records

Introduction

A service providing information on the changing patterns of work in a hospital should aim to satisfy both tactical and strategic management needs. The traditional approach to information services prescribed such indices as hospital occupancy, average length of stay by specialty and ward, average cost per in-patient case by hospital, etc. It is doubtful whether these statistics have been of great value at any level in spite of the regular demand for the figures by committees and the Ministry, and the time required to compile these statistics by conventional methods has left little time for the development of more useful forms of analyses. Furthermore, the daily management of hospital resources devolves largely upon medical and nursing staff who have virtually no basic information fed back to them regarding the past use of resources and the likely future demands.

In such situations, decision-making about the best deployment of resources becomes largely intuitive, and whilst in the past this may appear to have worked well enough, if hospitals are to meet the increasing demands for their services every possibility for deploying hospital resources to greater effect must be examined. The measurement of success or failure of changes in operational policies designed to achieve greater efficiency can only be made if information services are improved.

To supplement the basic hospital statistical data available for the Birmingham Teaching Group with information relevant to management and planning, an in-patient summary form designed for mechanical analysis was introduced several years ago. This system, based upon a record completed for each patient admitted (40 000 per annum), has been described by Hogben and Cross (2). Briefly, the information on the form was of three types:

(i) Personal, such as name, date of birth, place of residence, etc.;

(ii) Administrative, such as consultant in charge, dates of admission and discharge, source of admission, etc.;

(iii) Medical, i.e. diagnoses, causes of death, and operations performed.

The data collected thereon were transferred to punch cards; since 1958 these have been of the standard 80-column type acceptable to all computer card readers. The output from this mechanical system included:

(*a*) Tabulations of diagnostic and operation indexes for use by members of the medical staff;

(*b*) Data of interest to hospital administrators, such as distribution of in-patients with respect to age, department, duration of stay, place of residence, time on waiting list, etc.

A third category of use of such a system was provided by the introduction of the form into all the non-teaching hospitals in Birmingham at the beginning of 1965. Thus it is now possible to relate hospital admissions to a large known population at risk and various epidemiological studies with implications for planning future hospital services are being undertaken. Details of the scope and organization of the Birmingham study have recently been given by Mary Wall (3).

With the computer facilities which became available at the Regional Hospital Board in 1965, a routine feedback of information from this system to hospital administrators and medical staff was inaugurated. This is the basic objective of hospital activity analysis, as the term is currently used, viz. the supply of up-to-date analyses of the use of beds by consultant and specialty, by diagnostic and operation groups.

The Birmingham study, like most other studies in this field (1), is based upon a record which cannot be finally completed until after the patient's discharge and hence processing is

UNITED BIRMINGHAM HOSPITALS
QUEEN ELIZABETH HOSPITAL

REGISTRATION No. 737621		SEX F	WARD/DEPARTMENT WW3	NAME AND ADDRESS OF NEXT OF KIN
SURNAME HULBERTSON		CIVIL STATE M		P. A. HULBERTSON
FIRST FORENAME EVELYN		SECOND FORENAME MARY		S/A.
MAIDEN NAME SMITH		PREVIOUS SURNAME		
DATE OF BIRTH 110632		AGE 34	(CODE) RELIGION C CE	
DATE OF ADMISSION 010367		(CODE) 0	PLACE OF ACCIDENT	RELATIONSHIP OF NEXT OF KIN HUSBAND
(CODE) CONSULTANT 0717 PROF SLANEY		CATEG'RY 0 CODE	(C 'DE) SOURCE OF ADMISSION A WAITING LIST	TELEPHONE No. OF NEXT OF KIN NEW 1234
PATIENT'S ADDRESS 238 MAIN STREET--			OCCUPATION HOUSEWIFE	NEAREST POLICE STATION TO NEXT OF KIN NEWTOWN
NEWTOWN--			INDUSTRY	NEIGHBOUR: NAME AND TEL. No.
WARWICKSHIRE.				G.P.'s NAME AND ADDRESS
			DISCHARGE DATE	DR A B SMITH 127 MAIN STREET
			DISCHARGED TO:	NEWTOWN WARKS.
				TELEPHONE No.

Fig. 1. Spirit Master

entirely retrospective. No information regarding patients still in hospital is available for analysis, and the checking procedures with the follow-up of queries can delay analysis. This paper is therefore mainly concerned with an attempt to overcome these shortcomings as applied to patients admitted to the Queen Elizabeth Hospital, Birmingham, an acute teaching hospital of 641 beds, with a through-put of 15 000 in-patients a year. Predominantly, patients are admitted from waiting lists, as the hospital has no significant out-patient or casualty departments, these services being provided at present at the Birmingham General Hospital in the city centre.

Capturing data on admission

The medical records office of a hospital is the focal point of many documentation procedures. At the Queen Elizabeth Hospital a spirit duplicating process has been used for some years to produce, from a master stencil, various documents for each patient admitted. This master has traditionally been filled in by hand by a records clerk, either from a questionnaire completed by the patient prior to admission or by questioning the patient on admission. After a methods analysis of the various procedures involved, it was con-sidered practical to type the details on the master stencil, suitably redesigned. This decision opened up the possibility of producing data on punch cards simultaneously with the typing procedure, and

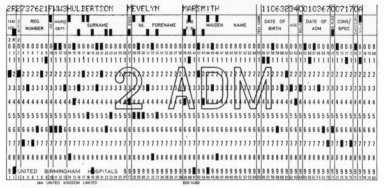

2ADM admission punched card

3ADM admission punched card

Fig. 2

after examining alternative machines, an IBM 826 typewriter card punch was selected.

By appropriate programming, the admission data of a patient typed on the master stencil (Fig. 1), are punched on to two punch cards (Fig. 2). The first card records all the administrative data except the address and the second card, which comes automatically into position after the completion of the first card without operator intervention, is used to contain the address. Each standard punch card used in the system is pre-numbered so that the computer can identify the cards as specific documents in the series.

The card punch simultaneously with the punching operation

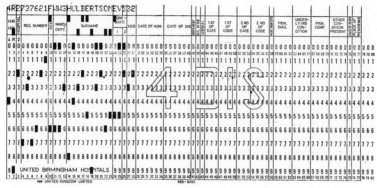

Type 1

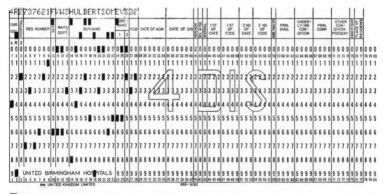

Type 2

Fig. 3. 4DIS discharged punched card

reproduces data in plain language form on the top of the punch card
and this information is checked against the questionnaire to ensure
that it is accurate. On completion of the checking operation the
spirit master is passed to a second operator and is used to reproduce
the clinical and administrative documents required. While this is
being done the punch card labelled 2ADM (Fig. 2) is reinserted
into the card punch by the first operator and is used to reproduce
the first 23 columns on to a card labelled 4DIS (Fig. 3). On this
particular card the length of surname is truncated from 13 characters to 10. The next 5 columns, i.e. 24-8, are manually punched
with the first two letters of the first forename, first letter of the

Computers in the service of medicine

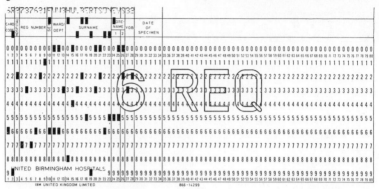

Fig. 4. 6REQ request punched card

second forename, and the year of birth. This card is then used to reproduce a second 4DIS card and also a card labelled 6REQ (Fig. 4).

After each admission, punch cards labelled 2ADM, 3ADM, and the two cards 4DIS are separately filed in appropriate pigeon-holes within the Medical Records Office. The punch card labelled 6REQ is filed with the patient's case-notes, a folder having been designed to contain punched cards.

For ease of reference, the items of information recorded and the corresponding fields on these punch cards are given in Appendix I; and the rationale of the system of patient and record identification employed is discussed in the following paper. Special mention should be made of the 6REQ card, which is at present used as a request card in the Biochemistry Department (which has data-processing equipment). Its format is such that, with appropriate modification from column 41 onwards, it can be used in other laboratories and departments of the hospital. The potentialities of such a punch card as a means of transmitting information within a hospital are also discussed in the next paper.

This system is used for all patients, whether admitted from the waiting lists or any other source, except that for an emergency admission a questionnaire is completed by direct interrogation of the patient.

A number of documents are generated from the spirit master at the time of admission and in particular a two-part identification sheet (see Fig. 5). This form replaces the case summary card referred

UNITED BIRMINGHAM HOSPITALS

QUEEN ELIZABETH HOSPITAL

REGISTRATION No. 737621	SEX F	WARD/DEPARTMENT WW3	NAME AND ADDRESS OF NEXT OF KIN
SURNAME HULBERTSON	CIVIL STATE M		P. A. HULBERTSON S/A.
FIRST FORENAME EVELYN	SECOND FORENAME MARY		
MAIDEN NAME SMITH	PREVIOUS SURNAME		
DATE OF BIRTH 110632	AGE 34	(CODE) RELIGION C CE	
DATE OF ADMISSION 010367	(CODE) 0	PLACE OF ACCIDENT	RELATIONSHIP OF NEXT OF KIN HUSBAND
(CODE) CONSULTANT 0717 PROF SLANEY	CATEG'RY 0 CODE	(CODE) SOURCE OF ADMISSION A WAITING LIST	TELEPHONE No. OF NEXT OF KIN NEW 1234
PATIENT'S ADDRESS 238 MAIN STREET--	OCCUPATION HOUSEWIFE		NEAREST POLICE STATION TO NEXT OF KIN NEWTOWN
NEWTOWN--	INDUSTRY		NEIGHBOUR: NAME AND TEL. No.
WARWICKSHIRE.			G.P.'s NAME AND ADDRESS DR A B SMITH 127 MAIN STREET, NEWTOWN WARKS.
	DISCHARGE DATE		
	DISCHARGED TO:		TELEPHONE No.

THIS PART TO BE COMPLETED BY REGISTRAR

42. DISCHARGED AFTER

Investigation or observation only	TREATMENT				Follow-up only
	Operation	Radiotherapy	Operation and Radiotherapy	Other	
1	2	3	4	5	6

43. DISPOSAL

TRANSFER TO (SPECIFY)				
Pre-convalescent unit elsewhere	Convalescent Home	Geriatric or Chronic Sick Hospital	Other Hospital	Part III Accommodation
1	2	3	4	5

HOME				DEATH			
Discharged	To await further institutional treatment	Unfit for treatment	Self discharged	Reported to Coroner		Not reported to Coroner	
				With P.M.	Without P.M.	With P.M.	Without P.M.
6	7	8	9	10	11	12	13

44-46. FIRST OPERATION DATE   DAY   MONTH   47-50. FIRST OPERATION
DAY = 01 - 31
MONTH = 1 - 12

51-53. SECOND OPERATION DATE   DAY   MONTH   54-57. SECOND OPERATION
DAY = 01 - 31
MONTH = 1 - 12

58. MORE THAN TWO OPERATIONS : If more than two, give total number of operations :

59-62. PRINCIPAL DIAGNOSIS (1)   63-66. UNDERLYING CONDITION (2)

67-70. PRINCIPAL COMPLICATION OF ABOVE (3)   71-74. OTHER CONDITION PRESENT (4)

75. CAUSE OF DEATH : Code to above conditions, i.e. insert 1-4 as appropriate

OFFICE USE ONLY
76-77. PLACE OF RESIDENCE CODE

THIS COPY TO REMAIN IN PATIENT'S MEDICAL RECORD

Fig. 5. Diagnostic summary identification sheet

to above which was also kept in the case-notes until the patient's discharge. The purpose of this sheet is to facilitate the completion of the diagnostic and operation details of the patient on a document which can be detached and forwarded for coding and punching, and simultaneously on to a document which is retained as a permanent record in the case-notes. Separate identification sheets are generated for each episode of in-patient treatment.

At the completion of the day's admissions, the card-punch operator manually inserts the date of admission into columns 29–34 of one of the 4DIS cards and by inserting a separate programme drum reproduces this information in the same field of all the other 4DIS cards. This procedure is adopted because the 826 typewriter card punch does not have the facility of reproducing information from one field of a card into a different field of another card.

One of the punch cards 4DIS for each admission is filed separately within the Medical Records Office until the patient is discharged, and the second punch card 4DIS, together with punch cards 2ADM and 3ADM, is forwarded to the Computer Centre each day. The ADM punch cards are used as input to add the new names to the computer in-patient file and the 4DIS punch card is used for validation purposes.

Capturing data regarding internal transfers, discharges, and deaths

The in-patient file on the computer therefore contains full details of each patient admitted, and is up-dated daily. It remains to capture details daily of patients who move either within the hospital or who leave. This objective is achieved by a Bed State Control Form (Fig. 6) which is printed by the computer in the late afternoon for each ward giving details of the patients recorded as being on that ward. The sister then indicates if any patient has left the ward and his or her disposal.

Details of an internal transfer (or a change of category or consultant) are subsequently punched on to the punch card labelled 5TRANS (Fig. 7). The relevant punch card labelled 4DIS in the Medical Records Office is selected and columns 4–28 reproduced on to punch card 5TRANS. Columns 29–43 are manually punched into

BED STATE CONTROL FORM

UNITED BIRMINGHAM HOSPITALS
QUEEN ELIZABETH HOSPITAL

WARD W10

PLEASE COMPLETE THIS FORM AS AT 00·01 HOURS ON
THE REGISTRATION OFFICE BY 08·00 HOURS ON

AND RETURN TO.

SURNAME	FIRST	SECOND	REGISTRATION NUMBER	SEX	AGE	CAT.	CONSULTANT	LENGTH OF STAY SO FAR (DAYS)	TICK PATIENTS PRESENT IN WARD	WARD TO	TRANSFERRED DATE	DISCHARGED DATE	DIED DATE	HOME LEAVE	OTHER REMARKS
PATIENTS IN WARD AT 00.01 HOURS ON 01/01/67															
ABRAMS	GEORGE	LES	674537	M	35	O	SMITH-DAVIDSON	17							
ACHESON	TIMOTHY	ALG	674538	M	49	O	SMITH-DAVIDSON	09							
BERKLEY	RALPH	RIC	560937	M	27	O	PRITCHARD	99							
CLATTERIDGE	DAVID	NOR	739654	M	36	O	PRITCHARD	01							
DAVIS	LEONARD	GEO	575594	M	73	O	SMITH-DAVIDSON	26							
DAVIES	LESLEY	GRA	675932	M	21	O	SMITH-DAVIDSON	13							
DAVIS	LEONARDO	GER	746497	M	22	O	SMITH-DAVIDSON	07							
EDMONSON	GREGORY	CHR	673654	M	28	O	PRITCHARD	37							
FRANKLAND	CHRISTOPHER	JOH	685374	M	35	O	PRITCHARD	74							
GUNTHORPE	IAN	HEN	695635	M	98	1	SMITH-DAVIDSON	39							
HARROLD	MARTIN	FRE	732871	M	16	O	PRITCHARD	26							
INKFIELD	GEOFFREY	STE	659371	M	74	O	PRITCHARD	26							
JOSIAH	STANKEY	MAR	659372	M	24	1	SMITH-DAVIDSON	31							
KINGSMEAD	HARROLD	JOH	658743	M	27	O	SMITH-DAVIDSON	11							
LANCHESTER	STELLA		658744	F	38	O	PRITCHARD	C7							
LARKINS	PETER	DAV	667896	M	45	O	PRITCHARD	01							
LAWRENCE	PHYLLIS	MAR	646973	F	36	O	SMITH-DAVIDSON	54							
QUEREDO	BEATRICE	GRA	736542	F	82	O	SMITH-DAVIDSON	09							
SIMMONDS	MAY	SHE	757954	F	39	O	SMITH-DAVIDSON	07							
SIMONDS	JOHN	EDW	684932	M	64	O	PRITCHARD	10							
SYMONS	JONATHON	GRE	697541	M	86	O	PRITCHARD	15							
THEOBOLD	JEFFREY	JAM	678926	M	21	O	SMITH-DAVIDSON	36							
VENDLEHEIM	JOSEPH	KEN	796999	M	32	O	SMITH-DAVIDSON	02							
WEJNSTEIN	ABRAHAM	JOS	485738	M	37	O	PRITCHARD	06							
VEROS	KARL	ROB	574831	M	98	O	SMITH-DAVIDSON	37							
YELLOWLEES	MATTHEW	LUK	672911	M	102	O	PRITCHARD	01							
ZACHARIAH	ISAAC	SAU	672912	F	17	O	SMITH-DAVIDSON	02							
ADMISSIONS REGISTERED IN RECORDS OFFICE FROM 00.01 HRS TO 16.30 HRS ON 01/01/67															
ANDERSON	JACOB	FRI	778921	M	63	O	SMITH-DAVIDSON	00							
SCOTT-FITZGER	PAUL	JOH	778923	M	27	O	SMITH-DAVIDSON	00							
MANSFIELD	IRENE	SYB	721654	F	21	O	SMITH-DAVIDSON	02							
OAKFIELD	CATHRINE	DIA	721676	F	25	O	PRITCHARD	01							

ENTER DETAILS BELOW FOR PATIENTS NOT PRESENT IN WARD AT 00·01 HOURS

HOME LEAVE (NOT DISCHARGED).

OTHER REMARKS e.g. CHANGE OF CONSULTANT, OR CATEGORY:

Fig. 6

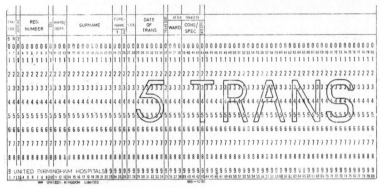

Fig. 7. 5TRANS internal transfer punched card

card 5TRANS with the date of transfer, transfer code, the new ward and the new consultant, and specialty codes if appropriate. The punch card 4DIS is then refiled within the Medical Records Office and punch card 5TRANS is sent to the Computer Centre and is used to up-date the information already recorded from punch card 2ADM.

When discharge or death is notified on the Bed State Control Form, the relevant punch card 4DIS is selected from the file, and the date of discharge and disposal manually recorded on the first card in each section and mechanically reproduced on to the remaining cards in each section. The discharge punch cards are then forwarded to the Computer Centre and the names of those patients are removed from the in-patient file.

Thus the Bed State Control Form is at once a computer output document and a punching document for input. It provides for the Computer Centre a check on patients bypassing the registration system, a means of notifying amendments to patient identification data, a record of ward and consultant transfers, details on deaths, discharges, home leaves, together with a summary of reasons for vacant beds. This system replaces the conventional system of records which most hospitals in this country employ, and has reduced the amount of clerical effort required from trained nurses.

Output from the new system

Several benefits in terms of reduced clerical effort and more accurate recording immediately accrue from the new system. Departments in the hospital are now supplied with daily bulletins listing alphabetically: (i) patients in the hospital as a whole and in each ward; (ii) patients discharged. A directory in alphabetical order of all patients admitted since the start of the system in April 1967, giving identification details, home address, dates of admission and discharge, etc., is readily available and is up-dated monthly. These print-outs not only reduce manual filing and searching time involved by records clerks, but also provide a more adequate index than hitherto with reduced possibilities of mismatching records.

The feedback of data to the medical staff is of a similar form to that previously mentioned as taking place in all Birmingham hospitals, viz., diagnostic and operation indexes, and analyses of the use of beds by consultant, specialty, ward, diagnostic, and operation groups. The latter analyses are still exploratory and will be modified after assessment of the response. An important feature of the new system is the form of control which has been introduced into the receipt of diagnostic and other data collected on discharge of the patient by the independent notification of discharge on the Bed State Control Form. Furthermore, there are good reasons to believe that the retention of a copy of the identification sheet in the notes, to be referred to on subsequent admissions or out-patient attendances, will result in more accurate specification of the medical data than hitherto.

Although not yet operational, an extension of the system to include patients on the waiting list has been devised. A waiting-list record card and corresponding punch card (1WL) has been designed (Fig. 8), and will be introduced shortly. This system presupposes that all members of the medical staff use the new record regardless of what individual system they choose to retain. However, it is anticipated that the feedback of information in several forms, alphabetical, chronological, and in order of urgency, incorporating details of data put on the list and provisional diagnoses, will encourage more of the medical staff to rely entirely upon a centralized waiting-list system. In addition to these listings of patients, this extension of the new system will provide opportunities for study of the scheduling of patients for admission and ultimately for predictions of the resulting work-loads on wards and departments.

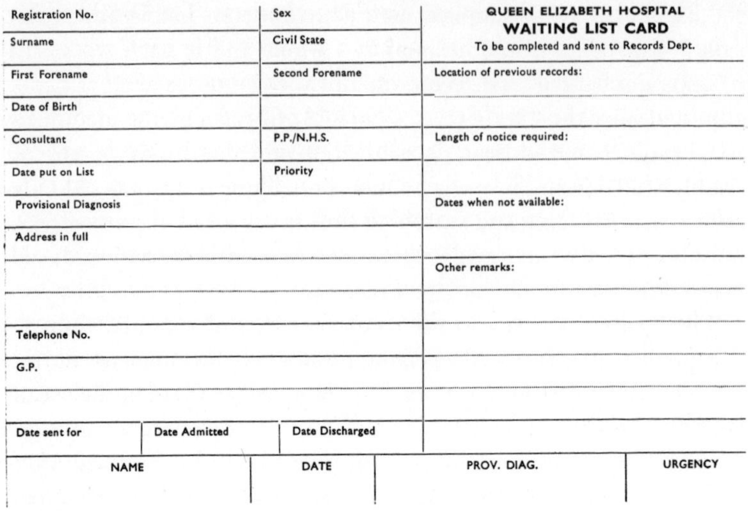

Computers in the service of medicine

Registration No.	Sex	**QUEEN ELIZABETH HOSPITAL**
		WAITING LIST CARD
Surname	Civil State	To be completed and sent to Records Dept.
First Forename	Second Forename	Location of previous records:
Date of Birth		
Consultant	P.P./N.H.S.	Length of notice required:
Date put on List	Priority	
Provisional Diagnosis		Dates when not available:
Address in full		
		Other remarks:
Telephone No.		
G.P.		
Date sent for	Date Admitted	Date Discharged

NAME	DATE	PROV. DIAG.	URGENCY

Waiting list card

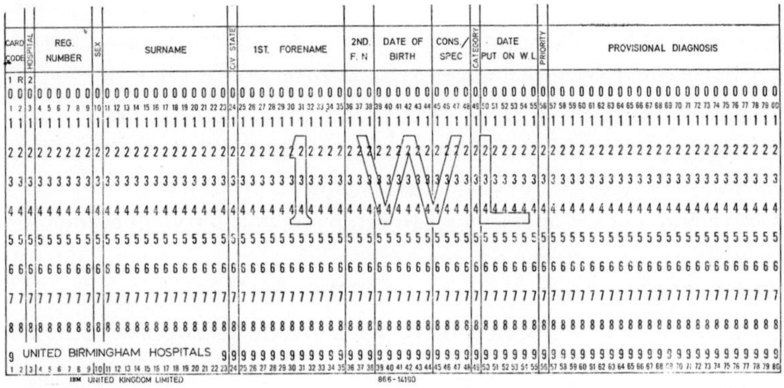

CARD CODE	HOSPITAL	REG. NUMBER	SEX	SURNAME	CIV. STATE	1ST. FORENAME	2ND. F. N	DATE OF BIRTH	CONS./ SPEC	CATEGORY	DATE PUT ON W.L	PRIORITY	PROVISIONAL DIAGNOSIS

UNITED BIRMINGHAM HOSPITALS

IBM UNITED KINGDOM LIMITED   866-14110

Waiting list punched card

Fig. 8

Conclusion

The foregoing outlines the developments in the field of routine mechanical and electronic processing of hospital in-patient records in Birmingham over recent years. The existence of the case summary card system and the experience gained over many years in continuing and exploiting such a system were of considerable value in planning the new scheme at the Queen Elizabeth Hospital. The Biochemistry Department at the hospital also had an automatic data-processing system in operation for some time (4), and early attempts at the linkage with the case summary records focused attention upon the need for generating patient identification data for use by several departments from a single punching operation. The 6REQ card initiated in the Medical Records Office at the time of admission is the central feature of the experiment. When other laboratories have similar systems to that in the Biochemistry Department, linkage of data from all such sources will be achieved by reference to the identification key which is reproduced on to all cards in the system.

Thus the short-term benefits of the new system are a simplification of hospital paper-work, reduction of transcription errors in identification and reporting, and the opportunties for producing integrated analyses of patient data. How far the latter can or should encompass the details of nursing and medical activity in relation to individual patients whilst still in hospital, has yet to be determined. Experience here and elsewhere has shown that detailed patient-care data can only be collected as a routine if they are obtained as a by-product of the usual recording procedures in a hospital rather than as a separate, retrospective, abstracting process. An experiment designed to examine the practicality and value of capturing data in this way has recently been started in the Medical Professorial Unit of the hospital.

Acknowledgements

The ideas in this paper and the succeeding two are the products of a team developing the project. The authors wish to acknowledge in particular the work of: P. J. Hills, computer manager, S. Sargent, senior systems analyst, and the Computer Centre staff; C. Faraday of the United Birmingham Hospitals Management Services Unit; and the staffs of the departments of Medical Records and Hospital Statistics.

References

1. BENJAMIN, B. (1965). *The Hospital*, **61**, no. 5. 221.
2. HOGBEN, L., and CROSS, K. W. (1960). *The Design of Documents* (MacDonald and Evans Ltd.).
3. WALL, M. (1967). *Medical Record*, **8**, no. 3. 13.
4. WHITEHEAD, T. (1965). *Progress in Medical Computing* (Proceedings of a one-day symposium organized by Elliot Medical Automation Ltd.), p. 52.

Items of information punched on to cards 2ADM and 3ADM

Card layout (card columns)	Field name	Length of identification fields (characters)
CARD 2ADM		
1–2	(card code)[1]	
3	(hospital code)	
4–9	(registration number)	
10	SEX	1
11–13	(ward)	
14–26	SURNAME	13
27	CIVIL STATE	1
28–38	FIRST FORENAME	11
39–41	SECOND FORENAME	3
42–54	MAIDEN NAME	13
55	PREVIOUS SURNAME	1
56–61	DATE OF BIRTH	6
62–3	(age)	
64	(religion)	
65–70	DATE OF ADMISSION	6
71	(place of accident)	
72–5	(consultant/specialty code)	
76	(category for PP, NHS, . . .)	
77	(source of admission)	

1. Brackets indicate the field contains necessary adminstrative information not formally part of the identification system.

Card layout (card columns)	Field name	Length of identification fields (characters)
CARD 3ADM		
1–2	(card code)[1]	
3	(hospital code)	
4–9	(registration number)	
10–80	PATIENT'S ADDRESS	

Items common to punch cards 4DIS, 5TRANS, and 6REQ

Card layout (card columns)	Field name	Length of identification fields (characters)
1–2	(card code)[1]	
3	HOSPITAL CODE	1
4–9	HOSPITAL REGISTRATION NUMBER	6
10	SEX	1
11–13	WARD	3
14–23	SURNAME	10
24–5	FIRST FORENAME	2
26	SECOND FORENAME	1
27–8	YEAR OF BIRTH	2
29–34	DATE, OF EVENT	6
35–40	(report number or second date)	

1. Brackets indicate the field contains necessary administrative information not formally part of the identification system.

3

The identification of patients and their records in a hospital

J. W. DALE
J. L. ROBERTS

Identification in a service environment

J. W. Dale, M.A., M.B., B.Chir.
Lecturer, Department of Social Medicine
University of Birmingham

J. L. Roberts, B.Soc.Sc., A.H.A.
Senior Research Associate, Department of
Social Medicine, University of Birmingham and
Statistician, United Birmingham Hospitals

The identification of patients and their records in a hospital

In a hospital the patient's records are used to control his daily treatment, and must be added to several times each day. The two basic operations performed on these records are that they must be linked together in a patient's notes, or departmental records; and they must be matched to a patient in a bed, or an out-patient clinic, or in the patient's home. In this matching to a patient, a hospital records system has an essential difference from research record linkage. Much of the published computer record linkage literature relates to the linkage of data for research purposes, but in this paper we examine the special problems of using electronic data processing to help in the record handling necessary in a hospital in the active treatment of patients.

There is an important distinction between the act of observation and the communication of the observation to others. We shall call the act of observation the *observation*, and the means of communication the *report*. The observations can be as different in kind as the reading of a patient's address, the measurement of a concentration in a laboratory, or the recognition of a clinical syndrome. Reports can be verbal and therefore transient; or substantial in the form of a written statement, a punched card, or a pulse in computer store. The first requirement of the report is that it shall not be capable of misinterpretation and consequently causing mistreatment of the patient.

In a hospital an observation can be made by one person who then makes a report. The message contained in the report may be interpreted by others who act upon its message. The *recorder* and the *reader* of the report are not always distinguished in scientific literature; both are often called the 'observer'. They should be distinguished, since different readers require different information if they are to act rationally (1). For example, a patient may be told by a nurse 'your wife rang', while the same nurse will tell the ward sister 'Mrs. Jones telephoned to inquire about her husband'. Both are reports of the same observation, but are constructed very differently. This distinction between recorder and reader is important in the hospital situation and has implications in the methods of handling patient related data which are demonstrated in this paper. Hospitals using the traditional methods of passing information by paper forms cannot use to the full the reports which have been made because often only a few readers can interpret correctly the information they contain. Often the recorder is unaware of all his potential readers, and since the wider his audience, the longer his reports must be, he resents any attempts to increase their usefulness in allowing correct interpretation to take place in new contexts.

The parts of a single report

The report of an observation relating to a patient consists of the following parts:
   a. The identification of the patient to which it refers
   b. Where the observation was made
   c. When it was made
   d. The quality observed
   e. The result obtained
   f. The identification of the report
For example:
129356 John Smith
Ward East Five
2nd October 67
Haemoglobin concentration
11.19.
Haematology number 593567.
a, *b*, *c*, *d*, and *f* can be regarded as labels to be attached to the result *e*. If there is only one single result, then we can regard this as the simplest form of a report and call it *one report*. When reports and

report forms are examined it is surprising how often the report lacks one or more of the above details.

Filing records

It can be useful to collect observations together in groups relating to the same time, or place, or quality; but it is well recognized that the most important organization of medical observations is with a *record* of all observations relating to the same patient. Therefore we must arrange that all observations bear adequate information to enable them to be grouped into those belonging to the same patient. We must also ensure that each observation refers *only* to one patient —a letter referring to more than one patient is unfileable.

File keys

Certain report labels have the property that they can be ordered. Words and numbers are examples. Numbers are defined as a sequence, and words have been assigned a sequence by custom. These labels can serve as 'file keys' to arrange a group of reports in an order. When reports are ordered on a file key they are said to form a 'file'. A file of reports has the advantage that access can be obtained to a single report in it without the necessity of reading all the reports. Similarly the patient records can be ordered, whilst themselves containing ordered reports.

Problems occur with mixtures of numbers and letters as in addresses, and with punctuation and special characters, since no universally accepted sequence exists for them. Even names cannot be ordered without some attention to special rules.[1] But with attention to these problems, by the use of punched cards and electronic data-processing (EDP) equipment the same patient-related reports can be arranged in several file orders using different labels as file keys. It is with this use of EDP equipment that we are concerned in this paper.

Access to a file

Two approaches are possible to find the location of a single report within a file; sufficient information can be given to assign a unique

1. See page 54.

sequence to the whole file; or reports may be grouped and share the same file position. With this latter approach unordered labels can be used to allow the programmer or file clerk to distinguish between the members of these small groups. If a computer is used to carry out the filing process, then whichever method is used all the labels must be file keys. Not to do so is equivalent to processing 'Hollerith strings' which cannot be analysed or compared without formidable programming. This may not be immediately apparent; but it should be appreciated that the computer cannot determine meaning, it can only match character by character; hence it is pointless to use labels for filing which could not be given an order in the computer. A filing clerk can use meaning, and could recognize the two labels '7 Corvedale Rd.', and 'The Cottage, 7 Corvedale Road' as the same.

Hospital patient record number

A patient record number is a label which can be attached to all reports about a patient within a hospital so that they may be grouped in a folder about a single patient to form a patient record. Traditionally space is allowed for a record number on every patient document; for it is the key on which the record officer orders his file of patients records, and at any time he may wish to fit a single document into that file. Since each folder of notes must have an assigned place in the file room, it is irrelevant to discuss whether other forms of number which give partial identification of the patient would serve instead. A record number exists as soon as the case folders are arranged on the shelves in a permanent order, and it has obvious advantages to write it down.

Report identification labels

Within a planned data system, however, all labels which serve as report identification assume a peculiar importance. We can present the information flow about a patient as a branching network of lines along which information passes from recorder to reader. At intervals in the system the information flow may branch to several readers who themselves may become recorders adding to the information already transmitted. This occurs at the point in a laboratory where a technician reads a request form with patient identification and diagnosis on it and adds to that form results from a laboratory test; it happens also in a medical records office where dates of admission and discharge may be added to an inquiry form from a Social Security office. We may call these branching points 'nodes'. All recordings made after a node has been passed can be linked conveniently if that node is identified. The event of initial registration of a patient at the hospital is one such node, each event of readmission another, each event of blood letting another. If these nodes and others in the system are labelled with the node number, the population of reports passing beyond each node is easily identified. Examination of manual data flows may show that the lines of flow have been numbered, not the nodes. Numbering the lines can be easier and it does allow the number of reports passing through the system to be counted but it does not allow the population of reports in the total system to be followed according to which parts of the network they have passed through.

PERSON IDENTIFICATION

Registration numbers, National Health Service numbers, or other code numbers at their best only identify the records and not the person.[1] They do not allow for matching a record to the person except by further reference to a cross-index of such record numbers and patients' names. Thus record numbers cannot be used for person identification.[2]

Populations

A recorder can only identify a person to a reader by stating labels by which he can be distinguished from other people. The most usual method of stating these labels is to specify a population of which the person is a member and then to identify him within that population.

1. Some types of numbers may have other serious practical disadvantages. Attempts to use the Midland Personnel Number (2) as a filing number in hospital file rooms in the U.B.H. proved impractical due to its length (10 digits) and the unpredictability of filing density at any point. These two problems were critical at the General Hospital which has over 500 out-patients a day.

2. It was considered by Hogben, at the time, an advantage of the Midland Personnel Number that whilst providing considerable specificity for record linkage it preserved the anonymity of the patient.

Obviously differing amounts of information will serve to label a person uniquely in different populations. We must know the size and nature of the population before we discuss the adequacy of a labelling system used to distinguish its members. A hospital records officer must distinguish in the population of the United Kingdom that special group of people who have been connected with the hospital, and since other organizations also have to identify sub-groups of the same United Kingdom population, the details they need are likely to be similar. If the details appear different in any particular case it is usually because a special population has already been defined. For example an education authority might distinguish only among the population of school age.

Populations in a hospital

Patients may need to be identified at hospital level from within the following populations.

1. The total population of the United Kingdom, not at one time but extending over the period for which records are to be kept.
2. The population of people who live in the hospital region.
3. The subgroup of the above who have registered with the hospital.
4. The population of patients currently under examination.
5. The population of in-patients on each day.
6. The population of all those registered as out-patients.
7. The population of persons on waiting list.
8. The population of any ward or department.

All these files can be maintained by computer. The National Census, and the development of record linkage studies have demonstrated this on a large scale, but the accurate maintenance of out-patient, daily in-patient, and ward files can also be tackled by computer methods. This could relieve the ward and clerical staff of much labour and has been attempted in the computer project at the Queen Elizabeth Hospital, Birmingham (3).

Labels available for person and record identification

It has been explained that if a patient's previous notes are to be made available on admission then a file of person labels must be constructed which also gives the patient record numbers. It is necessary to arrange the file of person labels in some order, and therefore labels which are file keys must be used, that is labels which by custom or definition have a sequence.

Such labels are:

1. Current names
2. Past names
3. Dates of birth, and of admission
4. Sex
5. Birthplace

The following are not useful as file keys because of variability in form of recording and because they change from time to time, but can be used as additional checks on record identification:

6. Address
7. Occupation
8. Title

The following are also used as 'labels' in hospital for informal communications about 'cases' rather than records:

9. Physician
10. General practitioner
11. Referring hospital
12. Diagnosis
13. Operation

There are other classes of labels such as photographs, finger-prints, and descriptions of physical peculiarities which are used elsewhere but are inappropriate to a hospital situation.

SELECTING RECORD AND PERSON LABELS FOR A HOSPITAL SYSTEM

It has been demonstrated above that an identification number is useful for record identification. File handling both on and off a computer may be made easier by it. But since most reports in a hospital must at some time be matched directly to a patient without recourse to a cross-index of names and numbers, each report must

contain a sufficient array of person labels to identify each person
within the populations commonly recognized at hospital level. How
this choice can best be made, the solution used in the University
Hospitals Project, and its effectiveness is now described.

We have said that before we can discuss the accuracy and adequacy
of such labels, it is necessary to define the populations within which
identification is to be made. We think that two populations must be
considered here; they are:

1. The total population of patients whose records are filed in the
   hospital, which we shall call the hospital special population.

2. The population of the United Kingdom.

1. The hospital special population

The need to identify a patient within the hospital special population
occurs more frequently than the need to identify him in population
2. In every acute hospital a report of an observation must be matched
to each patient perhaps twenty times a day. This occurs whenever
drugs are given, whenever a specimen of blood is taken, or a patient
is taken by a porter to theatre or an inquiry or report made about a
patient. In the Queen Elizabeth Hospital the report of the presence
of a patient in a ward is communicated on at least six lists each day
for distribution elsewhere in the hospital. Although an accurate
patient record number present on every document would be adequate for the Records Officer to link all reports within population 2,
it is obvious that most of the events mentioned above will require
matching the report to the patient without recourse to this number,
and the system must allow for matching by the least skilled members
of staff, junior nurses, porters, theatre attendants.

In choosing the right combination of labels for internal hospital
identification the population must be considered as the total population of patients whose records are stored or may be stored, in the
hospital, although only a small proportion at any time is under
active treatment.

2. Population of the United Kingdom

Identification of the patient within this population is required in many situations both inside the hospital and outside. It occurs at each admission of the patient; transfer of the patient home by ambulance; redirection of mail; follow-up report to doctor; death or birth notification; and whenever medical record linkage is attempted in the wider community. The labels chosen must allow use not only by records and medical staff, but also by general practitioner, telephonists, postmen, ambulance drivers, and the neighbour accompanying the patient. It is because of this variety of readers that the distinction made at the beginning of this paper between the recorder and the reader of a record has such significance in a hospital situation.

This statement of requirements makes it clear that name and address must be the essential practical patient-recognition labels for most of these circumstances, although the special requirements of research record linkage between hospitals will require file keys additional to name, if they are to be carried out by computer.

Address (and/or previous address) is a very useful label for person identification because of its availability and its specificity. For a prospective system the fact that it changes is of small importance: indeed this adds to its specificity. But for retrospective research projects it may be of little use as previous addresses may be unobtainable.

Table 1 shows the actual person labels accompanying samples from many hospitals sent to a central laboratory. This demonstrates another aspect of the problem of certain identification within the wider population—missing labels, and bearing this in mind a number of further labels may be considered.

It is because of current programming problems with address rather than because of any inherent weakness of it as a label for a prospective system that alternative file keys need to be added to name and address. Date of birth, inevitably a requirement of medical documentation, birthplace, previous surnames, and maiden name might be obtained from the patient, but are less readily obtained from relatives than are addresses. The Social Security number has the virtue of being relevant to an insured patient's financial interest when he is sick, but more than one person may depend on the same number (for example, Maternity Benefits). National Health Service

Table 1. *Person labels on samples sent to a central laboratory from many hospitals*

Label	Percentage of first 135 with details as first sent	Percentage of first 100 for which we now have details
Surname	98	99
Christian name	95	99
Age	74	97
Date of birth	15	97
Sex	79	99
Date of specimen	47	—
Hospital register number	24	86
Home address	27	97
Hospital	89	99
Consultant	93	99
General practitioner	—	94
Maiden name	—	93

It will be noticed how often age, date of birth, and address were missing when the specimens were received, although reference back to the referring hospital provided the missing details in nearly all cases. Usually about three of the items listed were given in any case.

The most frequent information recorded is the writer of the request (denoted by the consultant), and the patient surname and Christian name. Obviously surname and one Christian name are inadequate information in a hospital population, as the person most able to file the report is the writer, and not the hospital records officer. From our survey seeking full details it was obvious that the records officer was often unable to recognize the patient to whom the report referred.

number, which is universal but lacks importance to the patient, might be obtained less readily than Social Security number.

Files kept at regional health care record linkage centres need to choose from these labels such file keys as will still further subdivide a file ordered on full name. Once the keys have been chosen it is the construction of the file rather than its maintenance that is likely to present the major problem. For once a file exists for a region a relatively small number of new patients will appear each day who have not previously been admitted to one of the regional health care services.

The choice of labels in the Birmingham Teaching Hospitals Project

For this project it was agreed that all person and record identification items should be collected on registration of in-patients at the hospital; and that the computer input should be created as a by-product of normal recording procedures. In view of this the labels for identification within the special hospital population had to be a subset of those for identification within the wider population mentioned.

Certain further restrictions were imposed by the decision to retain the spirit master system for duplicating patient identification onto standard hospital stationery, including index cards used at the General Hospital which provides the out-patient service to the Queen Elizabeth Hospital.[1]

For identification of patients and their records in the population of the United Kingdom the labels have been chosen and are allocated to two punch cards, 2ADM and 3ADM.

For identification of patients and their records in the hospital special population, the labels have been chosen and card columns allocated to a card type 6REQ, and all the other internal report cards are of the same layout.

Card codes occupy the first two columns of every card used in the Hospitals Project. These codes identify card types and standard validation routines are used to protect each file from foreign data.

The computer-assisted patient records system has been implemented on a daily basis since April 1967, and is the subject of a separate, more detailed report (3).

The system may be extended throughout the 'balanced teaching hospital' centre site complex at Edgbaston, which will have many of the features of the future district general hospitals.

1. The use by a number of departments of IBM 870 typewriter card punches determined that the first 2 columns of each card have a card code, although this element of standardization incorporated in a general policy of standard card layout gives considerable benefits in the system as a whole. A small group is currently working on the design of suites of programmes to provide complex analyses of data recorded in the standard hospital patient identification format (6REQ type card) using one of several standard formats for results: (a) 10 fields of 4 digits, (b) 5 fields of 8 digits, or (c) 40 boulean fields, each occupying the 40 columns 41–80 of a standard card and others.

Appendix I to the previous paper (pp. 38–9) shows the card fields used for identification.

Conclusion

Hospitals frequently need to identify patients in the general population and this can only be by the use of names and addresses. The use of birthplace, date of birth, maiden name, and other esoteric labels is only relevant to the field of research record linkage. The list of labels used in the University Hospitals Project which allows for patient and record identification for active treatment and research is given. It departs from and makes more precise that given in the Tunbridge Report (4), which gave little consideration to the use of EDP methods. Linkage between hospitals, and the need for extra file keys is discussed. The construction of the file linking regional and national patient records to hospital records files is the major problem, and not its maintenance. It is obvious that considerable improvement in hospital registration procedures will be necessary if this is to be effected. The following paper demonstrates, however, that it is pointless to discuss how EDP methods can be used to link records nationally or regionally before the problem of recording observations is solved in hospital wards.

LENGTH OF NAMES

The choice of cards for input data to the computer assisted registration system demanded set lengths for each data field. Because the data might be used in future applications to send documents directly to a patient at home or to his general practitioner, it was desirable to reduce ugly truncations to a minimum without wasting computer time and space.

At first a field length of fifteen characters was set aside for surname and twelve for forename. The need to add more data in the remaining columns of the admission card encouraged us to measure the length of names in use. A survey of 1745 surnames of patients registered at the hospital indicated that thirteen characters would cover all but 1 in 10 000 names, and no forename of longer than eleven characters could be found in a dictionary of British forenames.

These field lengths were therefore set aside, and have been used in the system. No forename longer than eleven characters has yet been

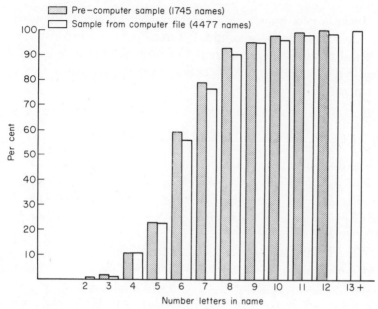

Fig. 1. Identification of patients by their records

found. Fig. 1 shows a comparison of the length of names on the computer file to those in the pre-computer system. The slight difference can be accounted for by the mis-registration of a small number of patients with double-barrelled names, in these cases the hyphen has not been excluded as it should have been, see Rule 10, Rules for filing patients' names.

The number of characters used in the parts of a name determine the file order of those names in any alphabetic list. As files become larger we shall not want to sort the whole file every time we merge fresh data into the master file. Ideally only one length of name should be used nationally in computer files, and we have suggested reasons for choosing thirteen letters for surname, eleven for first forename, and three for second forename.

We are compelled by the nature of medical records to use punched cards for recording reports about patients but there is not sufficient room for every punched card in the hospital to carry all these characters and hence our choice of a shorter length for internal cards.

In the hospital project whenever the computer is used to construct an alphabetic file however, the full name is used. Fresh data are merged by using the patient record number, and the other characters in the name are used to check the accuracy of the patient record number.

RULES FOR FILING PATIENTS' NAMES

Definition of a name

The Cataloguing Rules, published by the Libraries Association, lay down the basis of a definition of a name, to enable an ordered file of author's names to be maintained by a librarian. The rules assume that an order exists for any two names, or that they occupy the same position in a file, but nowhere is this order defined in terms adequate for a programme. The rules allow more, than one entry for each author to enable users unfamiliar with a particular form of author's name to reach the required entry by another route. It is unlikely that this multiple entry method will be immediately possible on a computer and we must therefore decide which form is to be accepted.

If record linkage is to take place by computer methods, then these deficiencies in the library rules must be made good.

To define an order of names, we have referred to the Birmingham Telephone Directory and endeavoured to give rules which will result in the same order as is contained therein. However, the rules for the order in the Telephone Directory are occasionally more complex than it is easy to programme. Where a change has been made, this has been stated. Usually the Directory itself indicates an unusual rule before using it.

Rule 1. Character set

A name consists of any of the following twenty-seven characters:

‘ ’, ‘A’, ‘B’, ‘C’, ‘D’, ‘E’, ‘F’, ‘G’, ‘H’, ‘I’, ‘J’, ‘K’, ‘L’, ‘M’, ‘N’, ‘O’, ‘P’, ‘Q’, ‘R’, ‘S’, ‘T’, ‘U’, ‘V’, ‘W’, ‘X’, ‘Y’, ‘Z’.

The first character will be called blank throughout the remainder of these rules.

The lower-case letters 'a', 'b', etc., are not distinguished from the upper-case letters.

The special characters apostrophe, stop, and hyphen are forbidden.

Rule 2. Collating sequence

The characters have an order called a collating sequence. This order is the order as given above, reading from left to right and down the page.

Rule 3. Parts of a name

A name is divided into three parts called the surname, first forename and second forename.

Titles such as Mr., Dr., and Lord, do not form part of the name.

Forenames in excess of two are not part of the name, and are to be discarded in the reverse order in which they are presented on the birth certificate.

Rule 4. Fields set aside for a name (*Modified Rule 24—Library Cataloguing Rules*)

Fields are set aside to store the parts of a name. The first field is the Surname Field, the second the First Forename Field, and the third is the Second Forename Field.

Rule 5. Field length

These fields are of a limited length. Two different lengths are in use in the hospital:

For external use	Surname Field	13	characters
	First Forename Field	11	characters
	Second Forename Field	3	characters
For internal use	Surname Field	10	characters
	First Forename Field	2	characters
	Second Forename Field	1	character

Rule 6. Justification within a field

The parts of a name are to be left justified within a field, truncated at the right-hand end if they exceed the field length, and padded with blank characters at the right-hand end if they are less than the field length.

Rule 7. Use of initials

If the field makes provision for more than one letter, then the part of the name should not be truncated to a single letter. That is, second forenames cannot be presented as an initial.

Rule 8. Missing forenames

If the person has no second forename, the field must be left blank.

Rule 9. Unused forenames (*Modified Rule 28—Library Cataloguing Rules*)

The forenames are to be given in the order recorded on the birth certificate, and not in the order of usage.

Rule 10. Compound surnames (*Modified Rule 25—Library Cataloguing Rules*)

Compound surnames are to be entered under the first part of the surname. Neither a hyphen character nor a blank character are to be used to separate the parts of a surname, which are to be closed up.
    Usage is not to alter this rule.
Thus:

Harvington Smith — HARVINGTONSMITH

Rule 11. Surname with prefix (*Modified Rule 26—Library Cataloguing Rules*)

Surnames of any national origin with prefixes of the following characters are not to have the parts separated by a hyphen but are to be entered as shown.

	Prefix	Surname	Entered as
English	A'	A'Bear	ABEAR
	Ap	Ap John	APJOHN
	D'	D'Costa	DCOSTA
	de	de Mille	DEMILLE
	De	De Morgan	DEMORGAN
	De La	De La Norgerede	DELANORGEREDE
	Le	Le Breton	LEBRETON
	Mc	Mc Donald	MCDONALD
	Mac	Mac Donald	MACDONALD
	O'	O'Connor	OCONNOR
	Van	Van Heuson	VANHEUSON
French	Du	Du Moncel	DUMONCEL
	La	La Rochefoucauld	LAROCHEFOUCAULD
	Le	Le Sage	LESAGE
German	Von	Von Hoffman	VONHOFFMAN
Italian and Spanish	La	La Lumia	LALUMIA
	Lo	Lo Catto	LOCATTO
	Da	Da Farina	DAFARINA
Dutch	Van Der	Van Der Haeghen	VANDERHAEGHEN

Note that some names have the prefix attached in common usage, and this will be maintained, e.g. VANDERKINDERE.

Rule 12. Compound forename (*Modified Rule 30—Library Cataloguing Rules*)

Compound forenames will not be separated into component parts, e. g. ROSEMARY not Rose Mary.

Rule 13. Unused forename (*Modified Rule 28—Library Cataloguing Rules*)

All forenames are to be considered and not only those in common usage, e.g. Arthur John Milton known as John Milton recorded as ARTHUR JOHN MILTON.

Rule 14. Forenames with variants

The original and not the variant form of a forename should be used. Not Droysen Hans but DROYSEN JOHANNES.

Rule 15. Nicknames (*Modified Rule 39—Library Cataloguing Rules*)

Before accepting any of the following as forenames, a check should be made that the original entry on the birth certificate is not as shown, e.g.

Jim (Jimmy)	JAMES
Fred	FREDERICK
Ted	EDWARD
Bill	WILLIAM
Bert	ALBERT or HERBERT
Tim	TIMOTHY
Sally	SARAH
Dot	DOROTHY
Pam	PAMELA
Beth	ELIZABETH

Note. A full list is being compiled.

Rule 16. File order (*Modified from the Telephone Directory*)

The names will be arranged in the order obtained by giving preference to the first letter of the surname field, then the second through to the thirteenth letter of the surname, then similarly for the forename field and the second forename field.

Rule 17. File Order for St. (*Reversal of Telephone Directory*)

This will appear in the usual file order and not out of sequence.

Telephone Directory Order	*Patient Directory Order*
Saint	SAINT
St John	STEVENS
Stevens	STJOHN
Stokes	STOKES

Further rules for names of immigrant populations, etc., will be available later.

ADDITIONAL RULES NECESSARY

Rule 18. Definition of maiden name

This name is the surname at birth, or as modified by an adoption order, and not any other surname previously used.

Rule 19. Definition of dates (*Modification of International Sanitary Regulations*)

Dates consist of six arabic digits. The first two digits represent the day of the month, the second two digits represent the month of the year, the third two digits represent the last two digits of the year. Preceding zeros are supplied in each part of the date field. Thus the first day of January 1901 is represented as 010101, not 1/1/1901, 1.I.1901, or any other form.

Century day number. For convenience all dates are stored in the hospital computer system as a day number, day 1 is 010101, day zero is 311200. Days of the nineteenth century are negative.

References

1. OGDEN and RICHARDS (1923). *Meaning of Meaning.*
2. HOGBEN, L., and CROSS, K. W. (1960). *The Design of Documents* (MacDonald and Evans Ltd.).
3. CROSS, K. W. *et al.* (1967). *Towards a Hospital Computer Service* (United Birmingham Hospitals and University of Birmingham Medical School).
4. Ministry of Health. (1965). *The standardisation of hospital records* (Tunbridge Report), H.M.S.O.

4

Patient identification on a regional basis

G.INNES
R.D.WEIR

Another experiment in identification

George Innes, M.D., D.P.H.

Lecturer, Department of Mental Health
University of Aberdeen

R. D. Weir, M.D., D.P.H.

Senior Lecturer
Department of Public Health and Social Medicine
University of Aberdeen

Patient identification on a regional basis

The two major uses of a medical record are, first, in clinical care whether this be the treatment of an individual patient, the development of diagnostic techniques to improve care or the evaluation of treatment and services, and, second, in research designed to increase knowledge, either clinical, epidemiological, or operational. The main common need for all uses of medical records is that of effective patient identification. If any records system is to become truly comprehensive then it is essential that all case records belonging to an individual patient can be linked together.

At the present time there are few hospitals which do not have a records system capable of linking together all records pertaining to one episode of treatment and most records concerning different episodes of treatment. But in many areas of this country the choice of hospital of admission does not lie with the patient or the referring general practitioner but is dependent on bed availability. Therefore a patient suffering a recurrence of an illness may have to be admitted to a different hospital. With the increasing complexity and potential hazard of many forms of modern treatment it will soon be essential for the satisfactory diagnosis and continued treatment of such a patient that the medical records pertaining to his previous admission be easily and rapidly available.

One of the important factors in determining the feasibility and scope of record linkage is the frequency with which patients change their address. At the 1961 census 18 per cent of the population of the city of Aberdeen had stayed at their present address for less than two years. Nevertheless, one of the advantages in the north-east of Scotland is that people do not move far. In 1961, 85 per cent of the persons resident in the Hospital Board Region were born within the area, and a further 9 per cent within the rest of Scotland. Therefore, to ensure continuity of treatment and facilitate investigative and diagnostic procedures there is, from the patient's viewpoint, a great advantage in having a regional, in addition to a hospital, records system. To prove effective this regional system need only comprise an index containing sufficient patient identifying items plus the unit numbers at hospitals previously attended. Previous records can thus be located speedily. The details included could later be extended as far as a case summary of each previous episode of treatment. The greater the amount of reliable information available in the regional system, the greater its value will be to the patient and clinician.

Electronic data processing will in future be used to a rapidly increasing extent in medical records work. Before this can be achieved a great deal of basic work has to be done on standardization of the material contained in a case record. However, any innovation to facilitate computer storage must not inconvenience clinicians in day to day use of the records and, in fact, should show some benefit to the clinician. During the period of change-over there would inevitably be some duplication of storage which, it has to be acknowledged, would be more expensive than either the present or final systems. It would seem that the introduction of a Regional Index would provide an ideal first step in the development of a new concept in recording so that a large proportion of the information contained in a medical record can be handled by automatic data-processing equipment.

This paper describes a regional records system for the psychiatric services, and studies which have been introduced to facilitate regionalization and computerisation of the records systems of the North-eastern Regional Hospital Board (Scotland). To help with this work a Medical Records Liaison Committee has been appointed with the specific remit to advise the boards of management on the improvement of medical records in current use and on the introduction of new medical records procedures.

Psychiatric case register

Prior to 1963 the two main psychiatric hospitals and the regional psychiatric out-patient centre each had their own case record systems. This resulted in frequent duplication of clinical history-taking and investigation. In addition to these clinical considerations, research studies (Baldwin, 1; Innes and Sharp, 2) had demonstrated the need for, and the benefit of, an integrated records system.

Commencing on 1 January 1963 a case register was introduced for all the psychiatric services in the area covered by the North-eastern Regional Hospital Board (Scotland). This system, which has been fully described elsewhere (Baldwin *et al.*, 3), is based on one case record for each patient. This case record follows the patient from unit to unit and therefore continuously comprises a complete and up-to-date record of that patient's psychiatric history and treatment. Both patient's and clinician's time is thereby saved.

Identifying and detailed social data are collected routinely by trained interviewers at a patient's first contact with the service. Patient movement and clinical data are recorded for each move the patient makes from one service department to another. Carbon copies of the main forms have pre-printed coding spaces. From these forms the data are coded and punched into 80-column cards for computer input. At present the information is stored on magnetic film in a second generation computer unsuited to data handling and situated just over one hundred miles away. In spite of this, several types of analyses have been carried out. It has been used as an aid to clinical, epidemiological, and operational research. Annual patient movement tables are produced describing the use of the regional services as a whole by means of counts of both events and people. A breakdown of these by administrative groups, individual hospitals, and services is also made. Clinicians use the register data files not only for research inquiries (for example, the number of alcoholic patients seen by a particular psychiatrist within a year), but also for more detailed projects where additional clinical data can be added to that information already in the computer and various analyses produced. The register has also been used for producing control groups of patients, matched for age, sex, occupation, and other characteristics.

The next planned stage in the development of this register is to adapt the system for the more advanced third-generation computing facilities to be available in the region in the near future. This will be followed by simulation of records office index work at present carried out manually.

It has been agreed by all clinicians that this composite type of record system is a great improvement over the previous haphazard method. Although the quantity of information included on each patient in the case register is considerable, the number of patients is relatively small. A total of just over 15 000 patients have been registered since 1963. This represents about 3 per cent of the total regional population. Thus the major problem in setting up the psychiatric case register was not the volume of patient turnover but the standardization of information to be collected.

Development of a regional index

The case for a similar system to be instituted for all hospitals in the Region has been made in the early part of this paper. The immediate benefits may be difficult to see because of initial duplication of record work and increased cost. Nevertheless this is far outweighed by the ultimate benefit of individual lifelong hospital case records, rapid access to previous medical history, and increased research potential. Unfortunately the stage of ultimate benefit cannot be reached without passing through the preliminary expensive phase. Studies being carried out in this region are designed to ease the problems in the initial stages of setting up a regional master index. The initial problem in a regional index of all hospitals is the actual volume of patient turnover. Because this index in its first year would include 25 per cent of the population and would gradually extend to involve about 80 per cent, the amount of information must be kept to a minimum.

The possibility of starting a regional records index is being closely examined at the present time. It is planned that this office would be separate from, but closely linked to, the main records offices in the region. This regional office would accumulate identifying data on all patients seen in the regional hospital services. Although initially to be maintained as a manual system it would be designed from the start to permit easy transfer to computer handling in the future. In addition a service would be provided by informing records offices of contacts of their patients with other units.

The initial problem is, then, one of accurate patient identification, which is the essential component of any comprehensive records system. Once the system of identification is operational then additional information such as dates of treatment, diagnoses, and case summaries can be grafted on as standardization of these items is achieved. These latter items can only be of value, however, when a satisfactory identification of the patient, and linkage with previous records is guaranteed.

In the majority of cases identification can be made by means of present surname, Christian names, and address. The likelihood of difficulties arising increases with the time since previous admission when items such as address (as mentioned earlier) and surname (in the case of married women) may have changed. In a small manual system additional clues may be obtained by patient's age and marital status, occupation, general practitioner's name, and knowledge of dates of previous admissions. When dealing with large numbers of patients these clues are insufficient. Items used for identification should ideally be those which are lifelong—surname at birth, Christian names, date and place of birth, and mother's maiden surname. Acheson (4) in an excellent and comprehensive discussion of the values of these factors, discusses the importance of giving weighted importance to these items. For example, there was an error of 3 per cent in recording dates of birth, but, for the year of birth, the error is more likely to be plus or minus one year than ten years or more. In describing Newcombe's work in Canada which had shown that, in conjunction with surname at birth, mother's maiden name was most valuable in patient identification, Acheson doubted whether it would be possible to satisfactorily record mother's maiden name in hospital records in this country. In a study of 114 000 Canadian marriage certificates it was found that these two items combined were unique in 80 per cent of cases. Mother's maiden surname has been collected routinely without

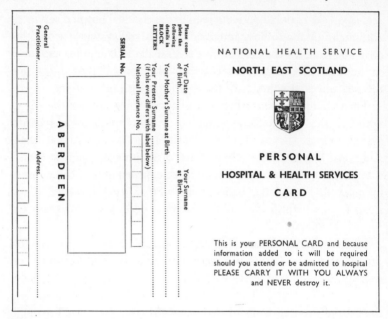

Fig. 1

difficulty in the psychiatric services here for over three years. Recent trial introduction into the general hospital records office met initially with some doubt in the minds of the records clerks as to why it was being asked. Explanation on this point has resulted in almost 100 per cent response from patients.

Acheson (4) also discusses the advantages of each patient having a unique identifying number as in many Scandinavian countries. In Great Britain all the population have a unique number, the National Health Service number, but this is requested only, for example, when receiving dental treatment. Only a small proportion of the public know their number, it being frequently confused with the National Insurance number. Also because of its varied letter-figure form the National Health Service number is unsuitable for use with data-processing equipment.

Card-carrying scheme
A project to discover whether members of the general population

	DISEASE	THERAPY	
Diseases requiring Replacement Therapy or Special Long-Term Management			**To be completed by Medical or Hospital Staff** Please enter Disease and Therapy
BLOOD GROUP				**DRUG SENSITIVITY AND ALLERGY**
IMMUNISATION			

To be completed ONLY by the HOSPITAL concerned :

National Health Service No.	
N.E. Region P. S.	A. G. H. and R. A. H. S. C.
Maternity Services	
	Other Services Please specify

Fig. 2

could be encouraged to carry a card containing identifying information has been launched. It was considered the benefits of card-carrying would be twofold. Firstly, positive identification depends on the patient giving the required information accurately. Accurate recall is synonymous with presenting a card containing these data. Secondly, only those persons not carrying a card would require matching by computer. If the proportion of non-carriers was small, then the demands for immediate access to the computer would be considerably reduced. If all patients have to be identified and matched using the computer then immediate on-line access is required. This is not likely to be available for some years.

In January 1967, cards (Figs. 1 and 2) were sent to all persons resident in the city of Aberdeen whose surnames began with the letter 'S' and who were included in the electoral roll. This comprised approximately 10 per cent of the adult (over 21) population. The card when sent out contained only the person's name and address and his number on the electoral roll. In addition to identifying information there was also space on the card for hospital unit numbers, drug sensitivity, and replacement therapy. The card was accompanied by a covering letter explaining the project and asking the recipient to complete the identifying data and to carry the card at all times. Publicity was also given to the scheme in the local press.

As from 1 February all records office and clerical staff in the area have asked patients with 'S' surnames attending as in-patients or out-patients to see their card. At this time as much additional information as possible is added to the card—hospital unit number and clinical data. Thus for patients re-attending with their card, not only is the hospital unit number immediately available for locating the appropriate case record but the unit numbers of all other hospitals attended are also available. This eases communication between the units concerned. A detailed questionnaire is completed by clerical staff recording the card-carrying habits of 'S' patients. Returns of all attendances by name, address, and electoral roll number, with reasons for non-carrying of the card, are made to the Records Research Unit who collate the returns from each unit.

In spite of the publicity attendant on the project only 50 per cent of patients carried the card in the first month. By the end of the fifth month the proportion of first attendances carrying the card had fallen to 33 per cent. An analysis of those attending in the first three months of the project has been carried out. During that period, from the sample of 12 000 persons who received the card, 1380 (12 per cent) attended a hospital on one or more occasions. Over the three-month period 57 per cent of all patients carried their cards, nearly two-thirds of out-patients, almost one-half of in-patients, but only slightly more than one-third of casualty patients. The proportion of card-carriers increased with the number of attendances so that 93 per cent of those who attended four times or more were card-carriers. Females (62 per cent) were more likely to carry the card than males (50 per cent).

It is not valid to extrapolate these sample findings to estimate the outcome of a similar national or even regional scheme where the whole population is involved. Certainly the findings do indicate that any regional records system dependent solely on card-carrying would probably not be successful. Nevertheless even at this level of acceptance card-carrying may have a place in the practical organization of a scheme of this nature. It may be that thought should be given to reducing the size and form of the card to bring it more in line with card systems designed for commercial purposes. An improvement in card-carrying would be desirable for although there is evidence that frequent demands for the card reinforce the carrying habit, it is, however, on the first of any series of visits to hospital that it is important for the required information to be available.

The card-carrying scheme was intended to reduce the amount of computer time (and therefore the expense) required in setting up a regional index. It would appear that, as stated earlier, computerisation of medical records will be expensive. But this will be justified when equated with the long-term gains that will accrue.

In this report some of the advantages and the difficulties which arise in setting up a regional records system have been described. The discussion has been limited to prospects in the near future (next three to five years) rather than the more distant future when linkage of all medical records (hospital, local authority, general practitioner, and vital registration data) will become feasible.

References

1. BALDWIN, J. A. (1963). *Scot. Med. J.* 8, 227.
2. INNES, G., and SHARP, G. A. (1962). *J. Ment. Sci.* 108, 447.
3. BALDWIN, J. A. *et al.* (1965). *Brit. J. Prev. Soc. Med.* 19, 38.
4. ACHESON, E. D. (1967). *Medical Record Linkage* (Oxford University Press for The Nuffield Provincial Hospitals Trust).

5

Computer applications in patient follow-up

J. CROOKS

How to keep track of the 'at risk' patient after discharge

James Crooks, M.D., F.R.C.P.
(ED., & GL)
*Reader in Therapeutics and Pharmacology
University of Aberdeen*

Computer applications in patient follow-up

The most important development in medical and surgical practice over the last two decades has been the advance made in therapeutic efficacy. The benefits of the proliferation of pharmaceutical products and surgical techniques have however been accompanied by a harvest of morbidity, in the form of iatrogenic disease, and thus the production of an 'at risk' population of ever-increasing size.

Much controversy surrounds the concept of the identification of 'at risk' populations in the field of 'natural' pathology mainly centred on the question of the economics of identifying large 'at risk' populations with a low yield of morbidity. For example, Sheridan (1), advocated that local authorities should maintain a 'risk register' of infants who, because of familial factors, pre-natal factors, difficulties at birth, and post-natal problems, were more likely than others to suffer handicaps, mental or physical. Oppe (2) has pointed out that stringent application of such criteria would mean that 60–70 per cent of all newborn babies were 'at risk' and points out that if such identification is to be of any practical value the group at risk must be a small one. Irrespective of the size of the group, limitation of medical resources demands that the yield of morbidity from an identified 'at risk' population must be large enough to justify the effort. Another important consideration is that effective methods of prevention or cure should be available at the time of detection of morbidity since otherwise the exercise changes from one of practical medical care to that of academic investigation, however worthwhile the latter.

From these considerations it follows that an area in which a

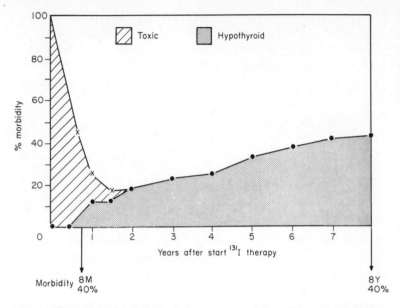

Fig. 1. The rising incidence of hypothroidism with time in 235 hyperthyroid patients treated with radio-active iodine

large return from the establishment of 'risk registers' would be obtained is that of iatrogenic disease. The extent of iatrogenic disease in highly developed societies is vast though not at present capable of precise estimation, except in specific instances. For example, it has been estimated that of the 100 000 patients with thyrotoxicosis treated throughout the world with radioactive iodine, about one-half will have become hypothyroid within ten years of treatment (Crooks, 3). Fig. 1 demonstrates this phenomenon of increasing morbidity (hypothyroidism) with time.

Another example is to be found in the late complications of gastric surgery, mainly for peptic ulcer. In spite of the well-recognized association of anaemia and bone disease with the post-gastrectomy state more than 30 per cent of patients have untreated anaemia, and 10 per cent develop bone disease many years after their operation (Crooks *et al.*, 4).

One of the main problems in establishing 'risk registers' in 'natural' pathology, the identification of the patient, is eliminated in the case of iatrogenic disease since the patient's doctor, whether in hospital or general practice, initiates the act (treatment) which identifies the patient as 'at risk'. In spite of this advantage, the high yield of morbidity obtained, and the relative ease of prevention or cure in many cases, it is remarkable that neither the hospital nor general practitioner services have accepted formal responsibility for tackling this problem. It is important, therefore, to seek the reasons underlying this deficiency in the medical services. They are to be found in the dissociation in time of the occurrence of the iatrogenic disease from the therapeutic act identifying the patient, in the dominance of curative over preventive medicine, in the ill-defined division of responsibility between the hospital and general practitioner services, and in the pressure of demand on available medical manpower. This is the dilemma of the 'lifelong follow-up' necessary if the consequences of iatrogenic disease are to be avoided. The hospital service, where the treatment responsible for later morbidity is often initiated, cannot cope with the logistics of the 'lifelong follow-up' of large numbers of patients for a variety of reasons including staff changes, clinical load, and organizational difficulties. While the population at risk is automatically divided, under the National Health Service, into smaller, more manageable units, within each family doctor's practice, the practitioner himself has not the necessary organization and often laboratory resources to take over the function. One solution would appear to lie in the provision of a system of 'at risk' registers and automated procedures using a minimum of medical manpower providing a service to both hospital and general practitioner in the control of iatrogenic disease. The operation of such registers with their dependence on data storage and linkage would appear to be ideally suited to the application of computer technology, and the following description of a pilot method of 'lifelong follow-up' is given to indicate one way in which this might be achieved.

Because of the high incidence of hypothyroidism occurring many years after treatment with radioactive iodine mentioned above and illustrated in Fig. 1 it was decided to establish an 'at risk' register

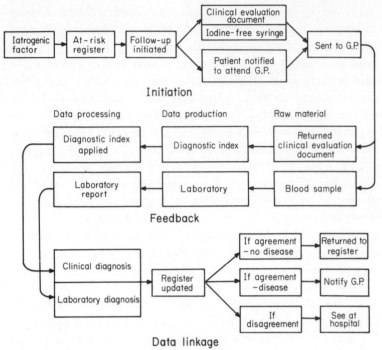

Fig. 2. Flow chart of 'automated follow-up'

for all cases in Aberdeen treated with radioactive iodine for thyrotoxicosis. Effective follow-up of such cases is of particular importance since the iatrogenic disease produced by treatment, hypothyroidism, frequently diminishes the possibility of the patient spontaneously attending the family doctor with symptoms of the disease. This is due to a number of factors including the dissociation in time from the treatment, the effects of the disease on the central nervous system, and the patient and her relatives ascribing the symptoms to the ageing process. The 'at risk' register was established in the following way. When treatment was given both patient and family doctor were asked if they would participate in the 'lifelong follow-up' scheme and agreement was obtained in almost all cases. The extent of this degree of willingness to partici-pate is of great importance since it signifies that both patients and doctors accepted the desirability of the procedure. Patients were placed on the 'at risk' register when the optimum results of the treatment had been obtained (the euthyroid state). The register consisted of a series of data cards containing information identifying patient, family doctor, clinical state at the last hospital visit, and details of treatment. Each year a card (patient) was raised mechanically by a secretary and this triggered a series of operations which are illustrated in Fig. 2. The initial operation consisted of the patient being notified to attend her family doctor and the doctor being sent a form with eight symptoms and six signs of hypothyroidism together with the criteria for identifying these features. The form is shown in Fig. 3 and was accompanied by an iodine-free syringe for a blood sample to be obtained. The doctor could carry out this investigation in under five minutes for each patient. The form and blood sample were returned to the secretary for processing. In the case of the form she allocated pre-determined numbers (discriminant functions) to each clinical feature and obtained a diagnostic score with ranges in which hypothyroidism should be suspected (Billewicz *et al.*, 5). The laboratory processed the blood sample and produced a measurement of the serum protein bound iodine which could be interpreted in the light of an established normal range of values. On the basis of this information the secretary could carry out an act of 'diagnosis' in which the 'at risk' patient could be classified by agreement of clinical and laboratory evidence, as normal (euthyroid) or abnormal (hypothyroid) or because of conflict between clinical and laboratory evidence, as suspected of the disease (hypothyroid). Those patients classified as euthyroid were returned to the register and the doctor and patient informed of the result. Treatment was initiated for the hypothyroid group, and further investigation arranged for the 'suspected' group at the hospital clinic. In the pilot study carried out in Aberdeen the 'at risk' register consisted of 223 patients treated with radioactive iodine for thyrotoxicosis who at the time of treatment were at risk of developing hypothyroidism some time in the future. These 202 patients were under the care of 155 general practitioners of whom only 9 did not co-operate in the scheme (94 per cent co-operation).

At the time of going to press 102 of these patients have already been identified as having developed hypothyroidism and

HYPOTHYROIDISM—DIAGNOSTIC INDEX

Name .... Age .... Sex ....

Unit no. .... Hospital ....

Observer .... Date.......................................

Previous anti-thyroid therapy: Type................... Dates.......................

SYMPTOMS (of recent onset)	DESCRIPTION	SCORE (Ring appropriate value) Present	Absent	Doubtful
1. Diminished sweating	Sweating in a warm room or centrally heated hall	+ 6	−2	o
2. Dry skin	Dryness of skin noticed spontaneously or on removing clothing, requiring skin cream	+ 3	−6	o
3. Cold intolerance	Preference for a warm room, extra clothing or bed clothing	+ 4	−5	o
4. Weight increase	Recorded increase in weight; tightness of clothing	+ 1	−1	o
5. Constipation	Bowel habits; use of laxative	+ 2	−1	o
6. Hoarseness of voice	Speaking voice; singing voice	+ 5	−6	o
7. Paraesthesiae	Subjective sensations of numbness, tingling, etc.	+ 5	−4	o
8. Deafness	Progressive impairment of hearing	+ 2	o	o
SIGNS				
9. Slow movements	Observe patient removing and replacing a buttoned garment	+11	−3	o
10. Coarse skin	Examine hands, forearms, elbows for roughness and thickening of skin	+ 7	−7	o
11. Cold skin	Compare temperature of examiner's and patient's hands	+ 3	−2	o
12. Periorbital puffiness	Should obscure curve of malar bone	+ 4	−6	o
13. Slow pulse rate	Count over 30 seconds Slowing present if under 75 per minute	+ 4	−4	o
14. Slowing of ankle jerk	Elicit with patient kneeling on a chair, grasping its back	+15	−6	o

Positive and negative totals   +   −
FINAL SCORE

Fig. 3. Questionnaire sent to general practitioners with scores (discriminant functions) inserted

are receiving replacement therapy with thyroxine but their follow-up continues under a section of the register designed to ensure that their replacement therapy remains satisfactory. Of the remaining patients 111 remain 'cured' to date while the detection procedure picked up 41 patients suspected of hypothyroidism. In 19 of these patients hypothyroidism has been confirmed and replacement therapy instituted (the automatic follow-up continues) and the remainder are still under investigation. Seven patients who have moved out of the area are being followed-up using the same system with the co-operation of their new family doctor. Allowing for the fact that at the time of the institution of the 'at risk' register there was a considerable backlog of patients at risk it is estimated that the hospital clinic work-load has been reduced to 10 per cent of that which would have been required to produce a satisfactory follow-up of these 202 patients based on the hospital clinic. This has been achieved by the expenditure of one hour per month of hospital doctor's time spent in supervising the register and by each general practitioner involved in the scheme expending less than ten minutes per annum in completing the questionnaire and obtaining the blood sample. Thus the scheme has been remarkably successful in Aberdeen and has resulted in a high yield of preventable disease which would not have been detected without careful hospital follow-up beyond the capacity of the medical manpower available.

The potentialities of this mechanical 'risk register' system in respect of computerisation can be readily appreciated on inspection of Fig. 2. Only by computer data storage, linkage, and programmed operations techniques could this system be comprehensively applied to the vast numbers of patients 'at risk' of iatrogenic disease in this country. Examples of patients who might appropriately be followed-up in this way are those who have undergone gastric surgery, or for whom chronic drug therapy including cortico-steroids and psycho-pharmacological drugs has been prescribed. Patients undergoing lifelong replacement therapy for the chronic anaemias, hormone deficiencies, and nutritional deficiencies of the malabsorption syndrome could well present variants of iatrogenic disease if they spontaneously stop treatment as happens not uncommonly.

A computerised facility of this type might well be organized on a regional basis and offered as a service to both hospital doctor and general practitioner. It would have the tremendous advantage of providing a measure of continuity independent of hospital staff changes and changes of family doctor (a common cause of failed follow-up). Updating procedures could readily be built into the programmes and linking such a system to other 'at risk' registers such as cervical cytology and diabetic screening could be readily attained. The way in which such a follow-up procedure would be facilitated by a computerised hospital record system is obvious.

The failure to apply available knowledge to prevent iatrogenic disease can be ascribed to three main causes. Firstly organizational defects in the medical services, secondly shortage of medical man-power, and thirdly a failure of communication. It is suggested that the application of computer technology would help to ameliorate all three deficiencies and furthermore would encourage the necessary re-unification of the hospital, general practitioner, and public health services.

References

1. Sheridan, M. D. (1962). *Mth. Bull. Minist. Hlth. Lab. Serv.* **21**, 238.
2. Oppe, T. D. (1967). *Develop. Med. Child Neurol.* **9**, 13.
3. Crooks, J. (1965). *Current Topics in Thyroid Research* (Academic Press Inc., New York), p. 1208.
4. —— Clark, C. G., Amar, S. S., and Coull, D. C. (1965). *Lancet*, **ii**, 943.
5. Billewicz, W., Crooks, J., and Wayne, E. J. (1966). *Proceedings of a Symposium on Computers in the Hospital Service* (Western Regional Hospital Board), p. 63.

6

A computer-based system for handling clinical data

F. KENNEDY
A. G. COX
A. I. M. GLEN
A. D. ROY
C. E. SUNDT

The first British system for an electronic clinical record

Frank Kennedy, B.Sc., M.B., Ch.B.
Lecturer, Department of Surgery
University of Glasgow

Alan G. Cox, M.D., F.R.C.S.
Lecturer
Postgraduate Medical School, London, W.12

A. I. M. Glen, M.B., M.R.C.P., D.P.M.
Medical Research Council
Clinical Psychiatry Research Unit
Graylingwell Hospital, Chichester

A. D. Roy, M.B., Ch.B., F.R.C.S.
Honorary Lecturer, Department of Surgery
University of Glasgow

Christopher E. Sundt, B.A.
Systems Analyst
English Electric Computers Ltd.

A computer-based system for handling clinical data

Introduction

A computer-based system is being developed to collect, store, and analyse current clinical data from patients who are receiving treatment in the University Department of Surgery at the Western Infirmary, Glasgow, and attending its associated peptic ulcer clinic.

This routine clinic has an out-patients session once per week, and on average forty patients, of whom five are attending for the first time, are seen each session. All of these patients have or are suspected to have peptic ulcers and are referred from general practitioners or from other departments. From this clinic patients are admitted to a general acute ward for surgical treatment and return for post-operative visits, being assessed thereafter at yearly intervals.

This clinic is accumulating information which could be valuable for research. Since peptic ulceration is a relatively benign condition and the post-operative survival after corrective surgery is long, analyses may have to be made on information collected over many years of clinical observation. In this type of clinical research it is not necessarily obvious now which items of information will require analysis in the future, and so it is essential to collect as much information as possible in a form suitable for analysis.

The clinic and department are primarily working units of a busy general hospital, and so any method of collecting information must be compatible with current medical and administrative practice, and must not increase the work-load of doctors or of other staff.

DESCRIPTION OF SYSTEM

General

A system has been devised to process this information using an English Electric KDF 9 computer. The system will handle the histories and clinical findings collected at the Out-Patient Clinic, the results of all investigations both routine (haematology, radiology, etc.) and special (acid tests) and details of operations, gastroscopic examinations, and the immediate post-operative course. Most of this information is collected by medical staff, some is provided by secretaries and technical staff, and a certain amount is obtained directly from the patient by the completion of questionnaires. The information is collected on documents designed for this purpose, and transferred to paper tape for input to the computer.

Documents

The documents have been designed to allow the collection of as much information as possible in numerical form. Numbers are used to record both intrinsically numerical information (age, weight, etc.) and also qualitative information which can be sub-classified into a restricted number of variables and can therefore be coded by numbers (sex, type of wound closure, etc.). English language words are used for qualitative information which is not easily dealt with by a coding system (symptoms, physical signs, etc.). These are coded by the computer with reference to a dictionary stored on magnetic tape. This concept is discussed later. The documents provide for most information to be recorded as single items, but lists of any length are used when the amount of information in a particular category can be expected to vary from patient to patient, for example, the number of previous operations. In some parts of the documents comment can be made with no restriction on form or content. One page of a typical document is shown in Fig. 1.

Most of the documents are completed by doctors during their normal clinical duties, which are already considerable, particularly in the Out-Patient Department. Within the system the surgeon is spared the necessity of writing out a history in longhand, and instead completes a document for computer input. From this

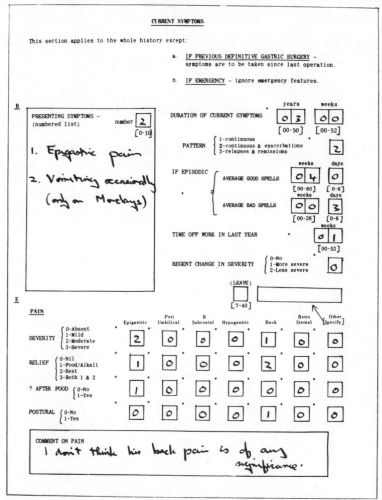

Fig. 1. A page of a completed document. * Indicates space for item modifiers (see text)

document the computer constructs a case history which is printed out on the standard hospital case sheet. To produce this the coded items are translated into ordinary language and the comments are transposed as they are written. These comments, although not readily capable of analysis, form an important part of the case history in the hospital records, and allow complete freedom of expression to the doctor collecting clinical information.

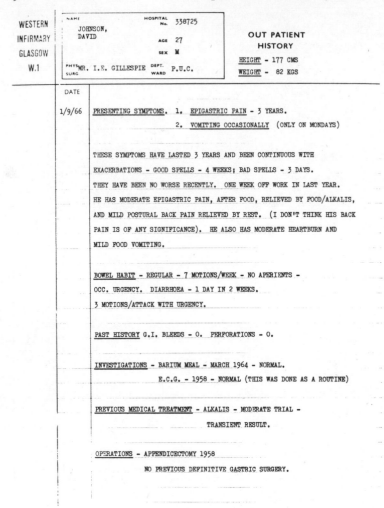

WESTERN	NAME	HOSPITAL No. 338725	OUT PATIENT
INFIRMARY	JOHNSON, DAVID	AGE 27	HISTORY
GLASGOW		SEX M	HEIGHT - 177 CMS
W.1	PHYS MR. I.E. GILLESPIE SURG	DEPT. P.U.C. WARD	WEIGHT - 82 KGS

DATE

1/9/66

PRESENTING SYMPTOMS. 1. EPIGASTRIC PAIN - 3 YEARS.

2. VOMITING OCCASIONALLY (ONLY ON MONDAYS)

THESE SYMPTOMS HAVE LASTED 3 YEARS AND BEEN CONTINUOUS WITH
EXACERBATIONS - GOOD SPELLS - 4 WEEKS; BAD SPELLS - 3 DAYS.
THEY HAVE BEEN NO WORSE RECENTLY. ONE WEEK OFF WORK IN LAST YEAR.
HE HAS MODERATE EPIGASTRIC PAIN, AFTER FOOD, RELIEVED BY FOOD/ALKALIS,
AND MILD POSTURAL BACK PAIN RELIEVED BY REST. (I DON'T THINK HIS BACK
PAIN IS OF ANY SIGNIFICANCE). HE ALSO HAS MODERATE HEARTBURN AND
MILD FOOD VOMITING.

BOWEL HABIT - REGULAR - 7 MOTIONS/WEEK - NO APERIENTS -
OCC. URGENCY. DIARRHOEA - 1 DAY IN 2 WEEKS.
3 MOTIONS/ATTACK WITH URGENCY.

PAST HISTORY G.I. BLEEDS - 0. PERFORATIONS - 0.

INVESTIGATIONS - BARIUM MEAL - MARCH 1964 - NORMAL.
E.C.G. - 1958 - NORMAL (THIS WAS DONE AS A ROUTINE)

PREVIOUS MEDICAL TREATMENT - ALKALIS - MODERATE TRIAL -
TRANSIENT RESULT.

OPERATIONS - APPENDICECTOMY 1958
NO PREVIOUS DEFINITIVE GASTRIC SURGERY.

Fig. 2. A case sheet print-out corresponding to the document in Fig. 1

A typical case sheet print-out is shown in Fig. 2.

Item modifiers

Clinical data which are often by nature rather imprecise must be
stored in an exact form in a digital computer. The concept of item
modifiers, described by Vigor (1), has been introduced to overcome

this problem to some extent. They are expressed by symbols which are associated with items of information on collection and thereafter are stored in association with them. They can be used by doctors to estimate the reliability of a recorded fact so that '75', '50' and '25' would indicate a probable reliability of 75, 50, and 25 per cent respectively. Some other item modifiers are:

'P'— Indicates provisional data and could be applied to a diagnosis which may be confirmed or otherwise at a later date.

'U'—Is applied when information is 'out of range' and is used when some numerical information is outside the normal range but is nevertheless correct.

'G'—May be used when a question is not answerable, e.g. menstrual history in a male.

Other item modifiers can indicate data which are collected retrospectively or missing data. Item modifiers will be of particular value during analysis when statistical weights can be given to items with different reliability ratings or the diagnosis is not accepted when it is provisional.

Dictionary

There is an obvious advantage in coding items of clinical information, but often the range is so large that coding by the doctor who collects the data is impractical. Such items include diagnosis, operations, treatment, symptoms, and physical signs. The system has been designed to allow the computer to handle terms in plain language and code them internally, and so removes the need to have a medically trained person in the time-consuming and unproductive job of coding the documents before input.

The computer will be provided with a dictionary of medical terms in five categories corresponding to those mentioned above, each category consisting of a list of names with all permissible variants. These variants are terms written by doctors, which, although using different terminology, are exactly or practically identical in meaning—for example, 'Pain in epigastrium'/'Epigastric pain', or 'Laparotomy'/'Exploration of abdomen'. The computer will match each term against the dictionary, so that a code number uniquely identifies it as an item in a category or a variant of it.

A dictionary will be devised initially by a member of staff, and the computer will add to this dictionary all new terms as they are encountered and print out a list of these terms. This list will be scrutinized by a medically qualified person who will instruct the computer to include new terms as names or as allowable variants in a manner which is medically acceptable. In this way the computer will itself assist in the building up of a dictionary of medical terms.

It will be necessary to keep a printed copy of the dictionary file so that when items are being extracted for analysis under their code number it is known exactly what information is being extracted. During such extraction it will be possible to use either main names or any variants.

Storage of data

Data are stored on two sets of magnetic tape—a patient data file and a dictionary file. The patient data file is built up by storing for each patient the data from each document as a separate record, and these records consist of several chains of linked items of information. The beginning of each record uniquely identifies the patient, and is followed by an indication of which particular chains are present and exactly where each begins within the record. This layout provides for easy access to any specific item of information, and since it is open ended permits expansion in the sizes and numbers of documents stored for each patient.

The dictionary file consists of a list of standard names held in alphabetical order within each category. Each name has an associated set of allowable variants also held in alphabetical order within the set. The names are stored in alphabetic form and each has an associated code number to identify it uniquely within a category and as a particular name or variant of a name. This is followed by a total of the number of occurrences of this term.

When a new term is encountered it is first held at the end of the appropriate category and remains there until an up-dating instruction places it in the acceptable position. The frequency of occurrence

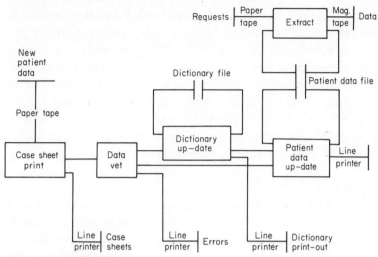

Fig. 3. Program flow chart

of new terms should gradually decrease as the dictionary file increases in maturity.

Computer programs

There are five specific programs which instruct the computer how to handle each step in the processing of data—case sheet print, data vet, dictionary up-date, patient data up-date, and extraction—operating as shown in the flow chart in Fig. 3.

The case sheet print program accepts paper tape input containing data from documents and prints out case notes from information contained on the out-patient documents.

The data vet program checks that data are consistent with each other and within acceptable ranges, and prints out reports on errors and on data which are rejected.

The dictionary up-date program alters the dictionary file according to any up-dating instructions and, by matching with the dictionary, replaces on the magnetic tape dictionary items with the appropriate codes. It also prints out lists of new terms added to the dictionary, and a record of the contents of any part of the dictionary when requested by a dictionary up-date form.

The patient data up-date program marries the vetted data with the items coded by dictionary up-date, adds these to the patient data file and prints out a list of all items added.

The extraction program extracts data from the patient data file according to criteria stipulated on paper tape, indicating exactly where the data are situated within the file. It performs simple arithmetic operations and writes the information on to magnetic tape in a form suitable for analysis by statistical programs written in Fortran, Algol, Usercode, etc.

Extension of the system

Although the system has been created for a particular job—to handle clinical data from peptic ulcer patients at the Western Infirmary, Glasgow—it has been designed with the possibility of extension in mind and, for this reason, the concept of 'general sections' within documents has been introduced. There are twenty-two general sections which have different groupings of coded items, of variable length lists, and of spaces for comment. The existing documents consist of various combinations of these general sections. The computer programs handle data on documents according to the general sections which are present, and so can deal with any new documents introduced, provided only that these are constructed from the set of general sections.

The general sections will have fixed ranges of values for coded items, maximum lengths of lists, etc., but when one is incorporated in a new document these ranges can be altered within wide limits if this is required. An illustration of two ways in which one general section can be used is given in Fig. 4.

Thus new documents can be introduced at any time to the system with no alterations to the existing programs, which means that the system can readily be extended to include further information or new research projects involving the patients in the scheme, and to include different data from other groups of patients. To extend the system to a further group, for example, another clinic, would entail considerable preliminary work to define exactly what information should be collected. Documents to record this information could then be constructed from the existing general sections.

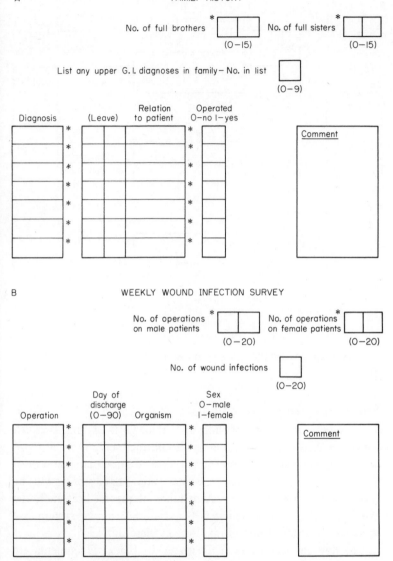

Fig. 4. Illustration of use of general sections

A. Shows how general section Y is being used as part of the documents. It consists of coded items, linked lists, and space for comment

B. Indicates a hypothetical use of the same general section for a completely different purpose. Note the changed range of values. Both layouts are similar to illustrate the point, but of course they need not be so

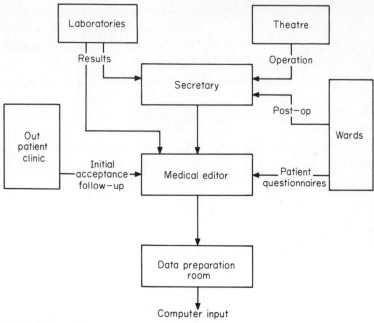

Fig. 5. Flow of documents

At this stage the system would immediately be able to handle this new data.

Administration of the system

The system will work within the framework of the Western Infirmary routine. In addition to the normal staff, there are two operators responsible for transferring data to punch tape, and until the programs are completely written and tested there will be two computer programmers. A member of the medical staff, the 'Medical Editor', has particular responsibility in the system but spends only a proportion of his time on these duties.

The flow of documents is illustrated in Fig. 5. Documents are completed by clinicians while interviewing and examining patients in the Out-Patient Department, by surgeons while dictating operation notes and discharge letters, by technicians carrying out acid tests and by the patients answering questionnaires. These documents are passed by the secretarial staff to the Medical Editor who checks that there are no obvious errors and adds a few code numbers. He also receives copies of results of investigations and codes these on to appropriate input documents. He passes all these documents to the operators who punch all the data on to paper tape using a Programmatic Flexowriter (Friden Ltd.). Errors in punching are minimized by using format tapes for punching and verifying. The paper tapes are then input to the computer.

Output material passes through this sequence in reverse order, the case histories being filed in the hospital records and the other reports reaching the Medical Editor for action. Out-patient documents are completed in the morning, edited and passed to the technicians for punching in the afternoon and submitted to the computer on the same evening. Thus case history print-outs can be available within twenty-four hours of interview.

Present position

At the time of writing (August 1967) the system has been completely defined and two of the five computer programs are at present being tested. Most of the documents have been designed and printed, and some are already in use to record information which will be submitted to the computer at a later date. It is planned to introduce the use of documents in the Out-Patient Clinic within the next month when case sheet print-outs will be available. Information has already been collected on over 700 patients on documents very similar to those that will be used in this system, and this information will be transferred to the recently designed documents to become available for storage within the system.

This position has been reached after at least three years' preliminary work by several members of the University Department staff with some advice and assistance from the Computing Department at Glasgow University. Since October 1966, when an analyst from English Electric Computers Ltd. spent two months on detailed specification, a member of the department has been occupied about 50 per cent of the time in developing this system. During this period advice has been frequently sought and received from the Medical Division of English Electric Computers Ltd. Since

November 1966, two programmers have been employed full-time in writing and testing the computer programs required, and for two years the department has employed two Flexowriter operators whose presence has been essential to the development of the system and who have also been occupied in recording information and in other specific research projects involving computer analysis.

The time-table for development of the system is up to schedule and plans to have the system in full operation by March 1968.

DISCUSSION

The ultimate role of large store high-speed digital computers in medicine is difficult to assess, but there is little doubt that their potential is considerable, and their widespread use in clinical data handling and in research will increase considerably in the next few years. The introduction of a computer system into a medical environment introduces many practical problems, and the recent literature reflects the fact that there are many more ideas than there are practical applications (Lipkin, 2; Waxman, 3) and this is particularly true in clinical data processing. In the United States preliminary work has been done by Schenthal *et al.* (4, 5, 6), Korein *et al.* (7), Slack *et al.* (8), and Ausman *et al.* (9), and a practical system for storage and retrieval of all clinical data obtained at a specialized out-patient clinic has been described by Levy, Cammarn, and Smith (10). In this country Bennett and Holland (11) have described a pilot study to determine the feasibility of processing certain aspects of case histories, but no practical systems to handle routine clinical data have yet been introduced.

Our system is designed principally as an aid to research, but at the same time it is producing for a limited group of patients up-to-date case records stored by computer. This obviously has important implications for future case record handling, and this aspect has been considered in designing the input methods, computer programs, and stores. In particular the concept of general sections from which documents can be constructed allows for extension of the system to other groups of patients. However, it must be emphasized that such extensions would require much detailed planning to define exactly what information should be collected and to control its accurate recording and transmission to the computer.

The flow of information from its source to the computer is the area where we anticipate most problems, and strict control will have to be exercised to minimize errors and loss of data. Some of these difficulties are well illustrated in a description by Baird and Garfunkel (12) of a system of electronic data processing of all records in a children's hospital. It had to be abandoned after six months of operation because of numerous difficulties, including errors of input and loss of data particularly by overworked or temporary medical staff, and the difficulty of integrating the system into the existing routine.

The development of methods of computer processing of the English language has important implications for the electronic handling of case histories. The introduction of the dictionary in this system is a limited step in this direction, and allows a certain amount of processing of medical terminology. Although more ambitious schemes for handling the English language have been devised by Baruch (13), these are on-line methods involving direct contact between the computer and the person collecting information which is expensive and time-consuming. Our method is a relatively simple one and the experience gained in its use will be valuable in designing any system for processing medical case records. Interesting information will be collected on the frequency of use of medical terms and this will be of value in future attempts to standardize medical terminology.

Our system of recording data will operate in parallel with the current medical records system, and is not an attempt to replace it. Much information, for example operation procedures and investigations, will be recorded both in a traditional form and on special documents for computer storage, and only in the Out-Patient Clinic, where clinician's time is at a premium, will the system, through the case sheet print-out, contribute to the hospital records.

Acknowledgements

We wish to thank Mr. David Vigor of the Computing Department, Glasgow University for many initial ideas, and we are grateful to

Professor D. C. Gilles of the Computing Department and Professor A. W. Kay of the Department of Surgery for considerable advice and assistance, and to the Hospital Services Department of English Electric Computers Ltd. for continuing help and support.

The Scottish Hospitals Endowment Research Trust and the Nuffield Provincial Hospitals Trust gave generous grants which made possible the facilities for data processing and the personnel for programming. Dr. A. I. M. Glen was initially in receipt of a full-time grant from the Mental Health Research Fund.

References

1. VIGOR, D., 'Machine Intelligence Workshop' no. 2 (edited by D. Michee) (in publication, Oliver and Boyd, London).

2. LIPKIN, M. (1966). *Gastroenterology*, **50**, 449–51.

3. WAXMAN, B. D. (1966). *Ann. N.Y. Acad. Sci.* **128**, 723–30.

4. SCHENTHAL, J. E., SWEENEY, J. W., and NETTLETON, W. (1960). *J.A.M.A.* **173**, 6–11.

5. —— —— —— (1961). Ibid. **178**, 267–70.

6. —— —— —— and YODER, R. D. (1963). Ibid. **186**, 101–5.

7. KOREIN, J., TICK, L. J., WOODBURY, M. A., CADY, L. D., GOODGOLD, A. L., and RANDT, C. T. (1963). Ibid. **186**, 132–8.

8. SLACK, W. V., HICKS, G. P., REED, C. E., and VAN CURA, L. J. (1966). *New Engl. J. Med.* **274**, 194–8.

9. AUSMAN, R. K., BAER, G. D., McGUIRE, M. R., MARKS, R. A., EWART, R., COREY, J., and WEST, R. L. (1966). *Ann. N.Y. Acad. Sci.* **128**, 1100–7.

10. LEVY, R. D., CAMMARN, M. D., and SMITH, M. (1964). *J.A.M.A.* **190**, 1033–7.

11. BENNETT, A. E., and HOLLAND, W. W. (1965). *Lancet*, ii, 1176–8.

12. BAIRD, H. W., and GARFUNKEL, J. M. (1965). *New Engl. J. Med.* **272**, 1211–15.

13. BARUCH, J. J. (1965). *Ann. N.Y. Acad. Sci.* **126**, 795–804.

7

Towards automated electrocardiogram interpretation

T.D.V.LAWRIE
P.W.MACFARLANE

Seeking a more reliable and available tool for diagnosis

T. D. V. Lawrie, M.D., F.R.C.P.

Professor of Medical Cardiology
University of Glasgow

P. W. Macfarlane, B.Sc.

Assistant Lecturer in Medical Cardiology
University of Glasgow

Towards automated electrocardiogram interpretation

The application of computers to the interpretation of electrocardiograms is relatively new and as yet techniques have not been completely perfected.

One of the earliest workers in this field was Caceres (1) who sought a method of analysing twelve-lead electrocardiograms based on conventional amplitude and time measurements. In effect, his group attempted to harness the computer to automate an established medical procedure.

On the other hand, Pipberger (2) approached the problem using vectorcardiographic methods, whereby only three electrically orthogonal leads are recorded simultaneously. Similarly, Stark and his associates (3) have, in addition, investigated the analysis of cardiac arrhythmias. These groups have used statistical techniques to obtain the most probable electrocardiographic diagnosis.

In other centres, computer assisted techniques are being used in research to increase the understanding of body surface potentials of cardiac origin and their measurement. Although not strictly computer analysis of electrocardiograms this may prove to be of considerable practical importance.

Gelernter and Swihart (4) have computed body surface potential maps using different anatomical configurations and equivalent cardiac generators while Selvester (5) has constructed vectorcardiograms with an analogue computer providing a system of equivalent generators. Body mapping is also being investigated clinically at present by Spach (6).

Reasons for automation

Computer analysis of ECGs has been attempted not simply for reasons of speed, since it is an established fact that where small computers are concerned, the method can be longer than a clinical interpretation which takes only a few minutes for a twelve-lead ECG. The advantages of this technique lie in the following reasons.

Firstly, each electrocardiogram will receive a more accurate interpretation devoid of observer bias than would otherwise be the case.

Secondly, increased numbers of ECGs can be analysed daily making it possible for one centre to undertake data processing for a group of hospitals.

Thirdly, the use of computers will eventually relieve medical personnel of routine ECG reporting and allow their deployment elsewhere.

For these reasons it was decided to establish an automated method of electrocardiographic interpretation for our own hospital with the further aim of extending this service to other hospitals in the vicinity.

COMPUTING SYSTEM

The establishment of a system for computer analysis of electro-cardiograms can be discussed under the following headings.

a. Selection of ECG lead system.

b. Recording of ECGs.

c. Preparation of ECGs for analysis.

d. Computer programmes for ECG analysis.

Fig. 1 illustrates the recording and computing system in schematic form.

A. There is at present no general agreement as to what constitutes the most satisfactory ECG lead system. Pipberger (2) suggested that a lead system should fulfil the following criteria: 1. it should enable as much information as possible to be recovered from body surface

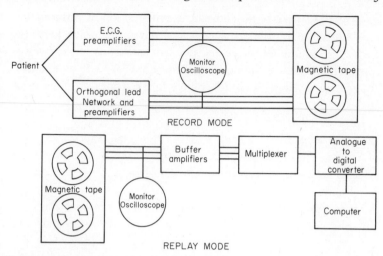

Fig. 1. Recording and computing system schematic

potentials; 2. the strength and electrical direction of the leads used should be consistent; 3. the number of leads should be as few as possible.

Some cardiologists who undertake computer analysis of ECGs use the conventional twelve leads (standard limb, unipolar, and praecordial leads). Others, however, feel that as much information can be obtained from corrected orthogonal lead systems (three leads) such as Frank (7), McFee and Parungao (8), and Schmitt and Simonson (9). One argument for using the conventional twelve-lead system is that duplication of present practices will be achieved as a first step in gaining the approval of physicians in using computer analysis. The validity of the interpretation is only minimally in question. Thereafter new criteria could be introduced. This is an approach which avoids the difficulty of persuading physicians that not only can computers be of use for ECG analysis but that an orthogonal lead system may be preferable for this technique. If a small computer, i.e. one with limited core storage of short word length is used for analysis, it is advisable that the amount of data utilized be kept to a minimum. In this respect the orthogonal lead system does appear to offer an attractive reduction in data (by a factor of four) and so a shorter time for analysis, whilst it is also

claimed that there is no clinically significant loss in information
(10). Furthermore, the orthogonal lead system, in which the leads
are recorded simultaneously and not sequentially as in the twelve-
lead system, offers a more quantitized analysis of ECG parameters.
In general it lends itself to a more mathematical technique of
analysis.

In order to obtain an answer to the choice of lead system both
the conventional twelve leads and an orthogonal lead system, that
of McFee and Parungao, chosen after a comparison of several
systems (11) will be studied simultaneously.

B. It is generally accepted that magnetic tape provides the most
suitable medium for recording and storing ECG records. In our
system, the recording of ECG signals is centred round a Hewlett-
Packard 3907B, seven-channel, six-speed magnetic tape recorder
which has capability for FM or DC recording on each channel.
Signals are fed to this unit from matching Sanborn 350 series
preamplifiers and a vector programmer which allows the production
of standard vector loops if required. This device could also be used
for twelve-lead ECG preamplification but is not as flexible as the
use of three separate ECG preamplifiers which allows any combination of three leads to be recorded simultaneously.

There is also a voice channel amplifier used for recording patient
identification. This will be quite adequate for research work but
will have to be superseded by a dialling code method for routine
ECG analysis.

A multichannel oscilloscope is incorporated into this part of the
system. This allows any four of eight inputs to be monitored
simultaneously before and during recording and during replay.

The tape-recording speeds vary from 60 ips down to $\frac{15}{16}$ ips, the
latter allowing signals with a frequency content of 0–128 Hz to be
recorded by FM methods. It has been stated (3) that the practical
frequency range of the ECG is 0.4–80 Hz which means that the
lowest tape speed would be acceptable. However, in practice it
seems advisable to record at least at a speed of $3\frac{3}{4}$ ips enabling
frequencies in the range of 0–512 Hz to be recorded. It is appropriate to acknowledge at this point that some investigators notably

Langner (12) have shown the value of high-frequency recordings in myocardial infarction.

The recorded ECGs can be replayed directly to a multichannel graphic recorder if desired. With the aid of a polaroid camera, signals can be photographed from the oscilloscope either during recording or later, on replay. Vector loops can be dealt with similarly.

C. In order that ECGs can be analysed by a digital computer, they have to be converted from their recorded analogue form into numerical or digital format. This is done by an analogue to digital converter (ADC) which is part of our PDP-8 computing system.

To satisfy the input requirements of the ADC the recorded signals are first replayed through buffer amplifiers which basically act as impedance matchers. The ADC then measures the voltage input to it and outputs the result in one binary word, having a switchable length of from 6 to 12 bits, i.e. the word can have a value in the range of 0–63 or 0–4095. A signed 11-bit number could be output alternatively, i.e. ± 2047 where the highest order bit denotes the sign. The number obtained can then be transferred from the converter to the computer memory and the process repeated at a rate dependent on the length of word desired (and the quality of the instrument). Ideally during the conversion the input signal will not vary and this can be ensured by the use of sample and hold circuitry.

The ADC can only accept one signal at a time and consequently to handle the 'simultaneous' conversion of multiple signals such as those of an orthogonal lead ECG a high-speed switching device has to be used to connect each channel of information to the ADC. This instrument is known as a multiplexer and in our system is also under computer control.

The conversion routine to sample each of normally three channels and store the resulting data is repeated every $\frac{1}{400}$ of a second, the time being kept by a computer-controlled clock. This rate, not to be confused with the actual ADC conversion rate of over 50 000 samples per second, was in our case determined by the initial computing system configuration and is intermediate to the rates used by other workers.

D. The use of computers for ECG analysis allows a large number of parameters to be tested for their diagnostic significance. Those which lead to an optimal separation between various diagnostic criteria will be retained in the final programme for routine use. In deriving such a set, the first step will be to separate the normal patterns from the others which can then be further subdivided into various categories such as myocardial infarction, ventricular hypertrophy, etc.

An Algol programme to analyse corrected orthogonal lead ECGs finds the various complexes at present by checking rates of change of vector parameters and starts with the QRS complex. The end of the T wave is then obtained but no attempt is made to find an $ST–T$ junction. The P wave is determined by an analysis of the data preceding that of the QRS complex.

A scalar analysis of each lead is then made, using reference points determined above, to find the amplitude and duration of the various P, Q, R, S, and T waves. At present no analysis of arrhythmias is available although this will be studied soon.

The remainder of the programme calculates time integrals, and selected vector magnitudes and orientations.

The analysis of the twelve leads, recorded three at a time, will be made using the same basic technique as outlined above. The approximate beginnings and endings of each wave will be found by 'quasi vector' methods and then the scalar analysis will find the correct wave durations, etc. This will avoid the necessity to write two separate programmes.

The output from the computer analysis consists of all the wave amplitude and duration measurements, vector parameters, and time integrals. A 12 lead ECG diagnostic routine is currently being tested.

Progress to date

A start was made to writing the Algol programme for ECG analysis on a KDF9 computer over a year before any of the PDP–8 system was delivered. When the basic system consisting of 4096 words of core store and the multiplexer–ADC became available it was only possible to use this system to convert ECGs to digital form and output the results for analysis by the KDF9 Algol programme. However, it was still thought advisable to continue with the Algol programme development since the basic routines might be of eventual interest to others even although each hospital will normally require a 'tailor-made' programme.

At present work is in progress on these lines with recordings being made from as many patients as possible. This has been facilitated by the recent addition of high-speed input–output equipment to the computing system. Other additions consisted of extra 4096 words of core storage, and two digital magnetic tape units for data and programme storage.

A start has been made to rewriting and testing the programme of analysis in PDP–8 language, now that the enlarged system has been made available, but this will be a lengthy process.

Discussion

With regard to automated ECG interpretation, there are many points of interest concerning not only our own approach in particular but the method in general. Those referring to the former involve problems of programming and satisfactory functioning of equipment.

The main problem with equipment has been the reduction of electrical noise to a minimum. This has been overcome but in addition a mathematical data smoothing routine has been included in the programme of analysis as suggested by other workers (2, 3).

Programming problems encountered so far relate to the Algol routines already written. Not unnaturally, these revolve around developing logic which will analyse correctly every set of data and not 90 per cent of the ECGs input. However, continual modification and testing of the programme will lead to improved performance.

The programming problems yet to be encountered are those of rewriting the logic of the Algol programme in PDP–8 machine code, with the aid of a symbolic language. The high-level language available for this machine, i.e. Fortran, is not presently of use for a large programme for many reasons, but this problem is probably common to most small computers where core storage space is at a minimum.

In practice, for example, accurate calculations in Fortran on the PDP–8 require that each number has three words for storage. In addition, various routines for multiplying, etc., have to be inserted in core store also along with the user's programme. Thus, with a small core store it is not possible to have a large Fortran programme. With machine language being used, as the only alternative when writing a large PDP–8 programme, particular attention has to be paid to arithmetical routines.

Another programming problem is that of the development of logic to analyse cardiac arrhythmias. It is possible to envisage arrhythmias for which it would be extremely difficult to write a diagnostic routine and as far as is known attempts at computer analysis of arrhythmias have not yet been completely successful. More recently it has been suggested (13) that a hybrid computer, i.e. a system with an analogue and a digital computer, may be of greater use in this respect.

With regard to computer analysis of ECGs in general, it must be acknowledged that the method has its limitations. It has been shown (14) that physicians can be more accurate than a computer in making certain scalar measurements but it has also been shown that they frequently did not give the same interpretation of VCGs when asked to review a set of tracings for the second time (15). Computer analysis should avoid this type of observer error, but will not remove the need for the physician to continue to understand the theory and interpretation of ECGs so that he can set out diagnostic criteria for the computer to use. He should also be able to interpret involved cardiac arrhythmias when required.

With increasing numbers of ECGs needing to be reported in hospitals an automated system of analysis does offer the advantage of relieving the physician of routine work. Such a system, however, is expensive both in terms of apparatus and staff (computer manager, programmers, technicians, etc.). To be economical it should be able to cope with analysis of ECGs from surrounding hospitals.

This in turn raises other problems such as transmission of signals from each hospital to the computing centre and the storage and printing of ECG reports.

Data transmission can be achieved by using a single pair of

telephone lines to accommodate three orthogonal leads, for example, each of which simultaneously modulates a carrier signal of different centre frequency for subsequent transmission.

Data storage would be necessary for comparison of an ECG with a previous report. This would require extensive digital tape backing facilities even for the reports of one hospital but if these were not available, the physician could simply compare two successive reports himself.

Systems in operation at present take about five minutes to analyse one ECG with up to half this time taken by output of results on typewriters. This time could be reduced considerably by the use of line printers, but these are expensive, costing more than a basic small computer. Alternatively, results could be output on paper tape at high speed for off-line printing. If it were assumed that the total computing time required for analysis of one ECG were then three minutes, it would take ten hours each day for 200 ECGs from a group of hospitals to be interpreted. It is apparent that, allowing a certain time each day for computer maintenance, ECG analysis in such a situation would occupy almost half of one day's computing time. Thus, there could be few other comparable tasks that one computer serving a hospital region could perform and this idea would appear to present considerable problems. It might be more advisable to have satellite computers in each hospital, linked to a larger regional computer.

Summary

Computer analysis of ECGs is still not a completely perfected technique. It is necessary, however, to assess its value now as computers will inevitably form an integral part of hospitals in the future. Although major problems still remain, it is felt that the more detailed analysis of large amounts of data will lead to increased accuracy of diagnosis and thus be of benefit to the patient.

References

1. CACERES, C. A., *et al.* (1962). *Circulation*, **25**, 356.
2. PIPBERGER, H. V. (1965). *Computers in Biomedical Research*, vol. I (edited by R. Stacy and B. Waxman, Academic Press), p. 377.
3. STARK, L., *et al.* (1965). *Ann. N.Y. Acad. Sci.* **126**, 851.

4. GELERNTER, H. L., and SWIHART, J. C. (1964). *Biophysical J.* 4, 285.

5. SELVESTER, R. H., COLLIER, C. R., and PEARSON, R. B. (1965). *Circulation*, 31, 45.

6. SPACH, M. S., *et al.* (1966). *Am. Heart J.* 72, 640.

7. FRANK, E. (1956). *Circulation*, 13, 737.

8. MCFEE, R., and PARUNGAO, A. (1961). *Am. Heart J.* 62, 93.

9. SCHMITT, O. H., and SIMONSON, E. (1955). *A.M.A. Arch. Internal Med.* 96, 574.

10. PIPBERGER, H. V., *et al.* (1961). *Am. Heart J.* 61, 34.

11. LAWRIE, T. D. V., and MACFARLANE, P. W. (1967). 'A clinical comparison of the Brody and Arzbaecher, Frank and McFee and Parungao Corrected Orthogonal Lead Systems', *Proceedings of the 8th International Colloquium on Vectorcardiography* (Vienna).

12. LANGNER, P. H., GESELOWITZ, D. B., and MANSURE, F. T. (1961). *Am. Heart J.* 62, 746.

13. AKAZOME, T., *et al.* (1967). 'E.C.G. wave measurement by a hybrid computer for automatic diagnosis of arrhythmias', *Digest of the 7th International Conference on Medical and Biological Engineering*, Stockholm, p. 102.

14. WORTZMAN, D., *et al.* (1966). *Ann. N.Y. Acad. Sci.* 128, 876.

15. SIMONSON, E., *et al.* (1966). *Am. J. Cardiol.* 17, 829.

8

Data processing in a clinical biochemistry laboratory

T. P. WHITEHEAD
J. F. BECKER
M. PETERS

Established and widening uses of a computer in investigating the patient

T. P. Whitehead, Ph.D., F.R.I.C.
Professor of Clinical Chemistry,
University of Birmingham

J. F. Becker, B.Sc., D.Phil.
Principal Biochemist, United Birmingham Hospitals

Margaret Peters, B.Sc.
Senior Biochemist, United Birmingham Hospitals

Data processing in a clinical biochemistry laboratory

Introduction

The use of laboratory investigation in the diagnosis and treatment of disease is continually expanding both in scope and quantity and the number of tests performed by hospital biochemical laboratories has doubled every four or five years during the last fifteen years. The resultant problems of laboratory organization are numerous, but three particular problems affect all laboratories. First, the transport of specimens and reports between the laboratory and clinic or ward; second, the mechanization or automation of the analytical process; and third, the handling of data within the laboratory. Although little progress has been made with the first problem, the second problem has received a considerable amount of attention which has resulted in the introduction of a large amount of mechanization in many hospital laboratories. The problem of data processing in the hospital laboratory is still the subject of experiments and this report describes one such experiment.

Data-processing techniques began to be used in the authors' laboratory in June 1964. The techniques were introduced for a fourfold purpose: first, to reduce the clerical labour of scientific staff in the laboratory and medical staff in the wards; second, to gain experience in data processing prior to the possible installation of a computer; third, to show that data in a computer-readable form was of use in laboratory management and patient care; fourth, to reduce errors in patient identification by communicating information in a machine-readable form.

During the last three years the techniques have been altered as experience showed how the system could be developed. At first, analysis of the data was performed on a card sorter, later we used a computer at a commercial data centre and since early in 1967 we have been using the hospital IBM 1440 computer. The equipment in the laboratory has not varied during this time and consists of an IBM 870 system which is a card punch with an electric typewriter link. The facilities of the system are such that at the time of punching a card all, or selected parts, of the information being punched can be automatically typed on the adjacent type-writer. In addition, by inserting cards into the punching machine, information already punched on the card may be typed to a selected format. The usual facilities for duplicating cards are also available.

DESCRIPTION OF PRESENT SYSTEM

The request for laboratory investigations

In the majority of the hospitals in this country, the doctor in the ward usually makes a request for laboratory investigation on a request form which gives details of the patient and also the test required. The patient's details may be written by the doctor or nurse and it is the experience of most laboratories that a great deal of the required information is either incorrect or missing. The 'Addressograph' system using pre-printed labels overcomes in-accuracies and the data are complete but transferring such data into a laboratory data-processing system is subject to error and is a manual task.

We are utilizing the data-processing system in the Registration Department of the Queen Elizabeth Hospital, where, when a patient is admitted, the details of name, forenames, year of birth, sex, registration number, and ward are prepared on an IBM 826 system. Request punch cards (Fig. 1a) are then mechanically generated from this master card, this is a simple task for the operator taking five seconds per card. Five cards are prepared for every patient admitted and these are placed in the patient's notes. This number of cards was decided upon after a survey of patient requests showed that this was the most economical and suitable number. On reachihg the ward these five cards are placed in a convenient rack adjacent

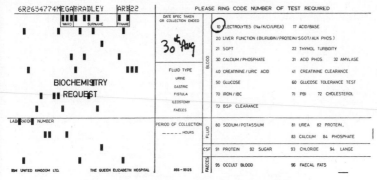

a. Front: containing patient identification, date and tests required

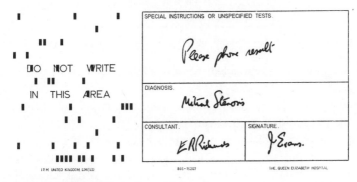

b. Reverse: additional information and instructions

Fig. 1. Biochemistry request card

to the resident doctor's desk where requests for laboratory work are written. Using one of these cards he is only required to 'ring' the appropriate test required as shown in Fig. 1*a*, add the date and then complete the details on the reverse of the punch card (Fig. 1*b*). This card contains the same patient identification details as the small wrist-band worn by each patient and the two are compared before blood is taken from the patient. On the blood specimen tube is written the patient's name, registration number, and date. The blood or other types of specimen are sent to the laboratory along with the punch card. On arriving in the laboratory a number is allocated to the specimen, this is written on the specimen and on

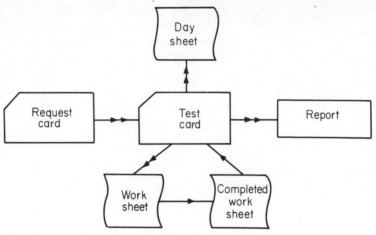

Fig. 2. Flow diagram of data transmission in the Biochemistry Department

the punch card, this is called the specimen number and begins at 001 each day.

Some patients have more than five laboratory requests and therefore need additional request cards in their notes. This situation is dealt with by specially marking the fourth card of the five originally supplied to the ward. When this fourth card is received in the laboratory a further five request cards are produced and sent to the ward so that they may be used for further requests.

Data processing within the laboratory

A flow-chart of the method of handling data within the laboratory is shown in Fig. 2. In this diagram a single arrow ($>$) represents a manual process, a double arrow ($>>$) a mechanical process. This data flow occurs in four stages as follows.

1. **Additional processing of the request card and preparation of the day sheet.** Immediately on receipt, the request card (Fig. 1*a*) is placed in the 870 machine and the first twenty-eight columns are copied on to one or a series of test cards. The punch operator adds the date and the test number of the analysis required. During this process the typewriter automatically prints a list of all specimens coming into the department on that day. This list, known as the

654774	M	BRADLEY	ARG	10.050	300867		
740853	F	SUMMERS	MA	10.051	300867		
737445	M	MASON	BET	10.052	300867		
737455	M	MASON	BET	21.052	300867		
737455	M	MASON	BET	17.053	300867		
7544211	M	KIRBY	ROJ	60.054	300867		
684381	F	CARTWRIGHT	AL	00.555	300867		AD
714533	F	HAMMERSLEY	JO	10.056	300867		
733546	M	WILSON	GEH	10.057	300867	2	
698831	F	OSULLIVAN	MA	20.058	300867		
598831	F	OSULLIVAN	MA	22.058	300867		
606112	M	NASH	WIH	10.059	300867		
606112	M	NASH	WIH	32.059	300867		
606112	M	NASH	WIH	70.060	300867		

Fig. 3. Part of a day sheet showing, from left to right, registration number, sex, surname, initials, test code, specimen number, date, sequence other than the first specimen, and miscellaneous test coding

day sheet, is shown in Fig. 3. It is displayed in the laboratory to act as a ready means of telling whether a specimen has been received and it gives laboratory workers information on workloads. The day sheet may contain additional information, for example, that a specimen is urgent or details of unusual tests which are not individually specified on the test cards by test number.

2. **Preparation of work sheet.** Depending on the workload, the test cards are sorted into test groups by hand or machine. The groups correspond to work areas in the laboratory. A work sheet is then prepared for each group. This work sheet is automatically typed by cycling the sorted test cards through the 870 system. The work sheet (Fig. 4) is collected by the appropriate laboratory worker and it is held in a loose-leaf notebook. The test cards are kept in the same order as the work sheet listing while the analytical work is carried out. Analytical results are written on to the work sheets by the laboratory worker on completion of the analyses, this being the only clerical task required of the scientific staff on routine work.

3. **Punching results into the test cards.** As the test cards are maintained in the same order as the work sheet listing, transferring

654774	EGA	BRADLEY	ARG	10.050	300867			*54*	*142*	*3·7*	*/02*
740853	WW3	SUMMERS	MA	10.051	300867	1		*42*	*136*	*5·2*	*94*
737⬤5	E1A	MASON	SET	10.052	300867			*375*	*,38*	*5·8*	*99*
714533	E2B	HAMMERSLEY	JO	10.056	300867			*123*	*141*	*4·2*	*104*
733546	WWG	WILSON	GEH	10.057	300867	2		*65*	*128*	*3·2*	*84*
606112	E3B	NASH	WIH	10.059	300867			*48*	*136*	*4·0*	*94*

Fig. 4. Part of a work sheet showing, from left to right, registration number, ward, name, test code, specimen number, date and manually entered test results

the results from the work sheets is eased. A visual check of the patient identification printed along the top of the card is all that is necessary before punching the results from the work sheet. Recording and punching results are manual operations and therefore subject to more error. Improvements to these processes, that is by mechanically calculating the result and automatically recording this in a computer readable form, is the next data-processing task under investigation in this department.

4. **Preparation of the report.** The report is typed by the 870 system from the completed cards which now contain the patient identification and the result (Fig. 5). The salary-slip type of report is used (Fig. 6) as it constitutes convenient stationery for use with the 870 system and provides economical and acceptable display in patient's notes. Many such reports can be attached to one mount sheet in a patient's notes and all may be seen without the turning over of several report forms.

The ten different coloured test cards are all of the same general format, each one corresponding to a specific report form.

APPLICATIONS OF COMPUTER READABLE DATA

It is important to emphasize that the computer readable data on punch cards is produced as a by-product of a data-processing

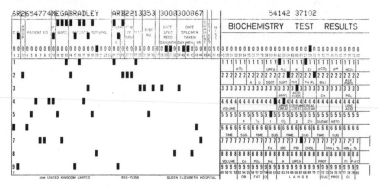

Fig. 5. Completed test card corresponding to the first line of the work sheet shown in Figure 4

system which in itself is worthwhile for the production of laboratory reports.

The IBM 1440 computer was installed at the beginning of 1967. It is a 16K random access machine equipped with magnetic disc drives and tape units, a paper-tape reader, a card reader and punch, and a line printer. Prior to the installation of this computer, facilities at a data centre were used. The present computer is housed some 200 yards from the laboratory and laboratory programs account, at present, for some three hours computing time each week. All programs have been written in Fortran IV with the exception of one project involving extensive file handling for which a commercially orientated language is more suited.

During the last two years we have concentrated on the use of the computer in assessing the accuracy and precision of laboratory results ('quality control') and in laboratory management techniques. Quality control of laboratory results is an increasingly important facet of laboratory management and maintaining accuracy and precision is an important aid to a laboratory head. The use of such techniques will be described and illustrated with the various computer output documents.

Quality control

Quality control may only be fully exploited by having data in computer readable form. For some six months we have computed

SERUM

65477 FGA BRADLEY AR G 10.056

DATE SPEC TAKEN   COMMENT PO_2 ____ mm. Hg

300867
DAY MO YR

	UREA	SODIUM	POTASSIUM	CHLORIDE	P_{CO_2}	pH	STAND HCO_3
	54	142	3.7	102			
	mg./100 ml.	m.eq.L	m.eq.L	m.eq.L	mm.Hg		m.eq.L

DATE SPECIMEN RECEIVED IF DIFFERENT FROM DATE TAKEN

COMMENT CODE
1. HAEMOLYSED
2. INSUFFICIENT
3. PLEASE REPEAT
4. SPEC. INCORRECTLY COLLECTED

Fig. 6. Report slip generated from the test card shown in Figure 5

CONTROL CHART – MAINLAB. –   14 : 3 : 67

ANALYSIS	DAILY MEAN	RUNNING MEAN	DAILY S.DEV	RUNNING S.DEV	CUSUM	NO. WITHIN RANGE	TOTAL NO. OF TESTS	VALUE POOL	CUSUM POOL	VALUE CONTROL
UREA	41.31	38.87	15.58	14.52	89.60	39	49	64.00	11.00	59.00
SODIUM	136.32	137.37	4.94	5.36	-40.47	47	49	140.00	-22.00	140.00
POTASSIUM	4.26	4.35	0.52	0.57	-2.31	38	49	4.40	-2.00	5.10
CHLORIDE	99.47	98.69	4.73	7.19	19.89	47	49	101.00	-22.00	101.00
PCO2	40.82	42.32	4.88	6.24	-64.67	11	14	0.00	0.00	0.00
PH	7.40	7.41	0.05	0.04	0.45	10	14	7.48	-0.07	0.00
HCO3	24.34	25.32	1.90	1.57	-11.02	12	14	28.70	-5.72	0.00
S.G.O.T.	58.00	46.55	36.71	30.05	-181.21	11	12	47.00	-45.48	15.00
ALK. PHOS	12.46	12.93	8.03	8.18	-20.75	18	18	10.80	-0.22	4.10
PHOSPHATE	4.69	4.05	1.51	1.44	7.37	15	16	3.50	-0.70	13.00
CHOLESTER.	224.50	223.12	52.35	57.28	-199.56	16	16	185.00	-10.00	0.00

(Column groups: T E S T   S E R A — POOL; SERA; CONTROL)

Fig. 7. Daily quality control chart

daily quantities which enable us to establish and improve the control of certain routine analytical determinations. We chose fourteen determinations as being most suited to this type of control and for each of these we compute:

    a. The mean value of patients' results—excluding in some cases results falling outside a specified range, for example, serum urea results greater than 80;

    b. The standard deviation of results about their mean value;

    c. A running mean which is the average value of the previous ten days' mean value. This quantity provides a basis for comparison of current and previous mean values;

    d. A running standard deviation—again the average of the previous ten days' values which allows comparison of current and previous population;

    e. The cusum of the mean value. This is a statistical technique by which trends away from a reference value may be shown. The reference value we have chosen for each determination is the mean value of patients' results for the previous year. (These techniques are fully described in the ICI Monograph No. 3 *Cumulative Sum Techniques*);

    f. The cusum value of the pool sera. The pool serum is analysed each day and is a sample taken from a large stock of serum. The reference value has previously been determined by calculating the mean of several determinations.

The values for each determinate are associated in a control chart (see Fig. 7) with pool and control values, the number of tests performed and the number within any specified range.

The chart is produced daily at 4 p.m. and includes data for any of the fourteen determinations performed that day. The running time for the quality control programme for an average day's data is approximately five minutes.

Previously quality control data were available on a limited scale only and generally not until the next day. An important advantage of having 'live' quality control data is that the validity of patients' results may be established before ward reports are issued and any appropriate action may be taken for those determinations not showing the necessary degree of control, for example, standards may be changed before the next day's analysis.

Fig. 8 shows the cumulative sum of both the daily mean and the pooled serum values for urea. There is an alteration in the slope of the daily mean cusum on 13 January which is not reflected as it should be in the cusum of the pool serum. This is due to a tendency of some technicians to maintain the known value of the pool serum. Misrepresentation of this value would—without the availability of live quality control data—disguise the fact that the urea test results were out of control.

Laboratory management

An area of laboratory management which can now be more thoroughly investigated is the analysis of work performed in the laboratory.

Detailed information about the type and quantity of determinations performed is of value in the planning of laboratory work. Such information is now made available weekly both in actual numbers and as percentages of total workload. The data is also held on magnetic tape so that variations and trends may be readily computed. It will be necessary to build up at least a year's file of data before detailed analysis is possible. Short-term analysis has, however, yielded much information which will be useful in laboratory reorganization.

Investigation of distribution of results

Fig. 9 is an example of a computer-generated histogram of uric acid values in male patients admitted to the hospital; Fig. 10 shows the corresponding histogram for females. The computer calculates the percentages of the total number of results in 0.5 mg/100 ml intervals. The line printer prints the histogram, and records the percentage of results above or below the values represented in the histogram. Mere inspection of the histograms gives a considerable amount of information which is of use in assessing the significance of results. For example, the accepted 'normal range' of serum uric acid is 2–6.5 mg/100 ml. The histogram shows that one in ten females

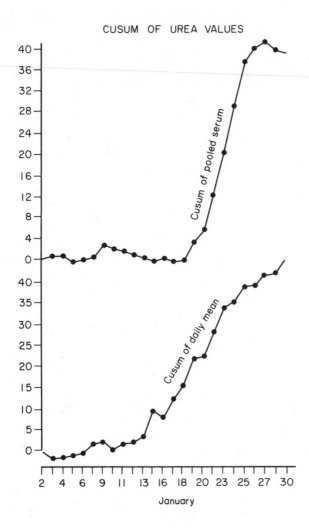

Fig. 8. Cusum of urea values for January 1967 showing a comparison of the cusum of the daily mean and the pooled serum

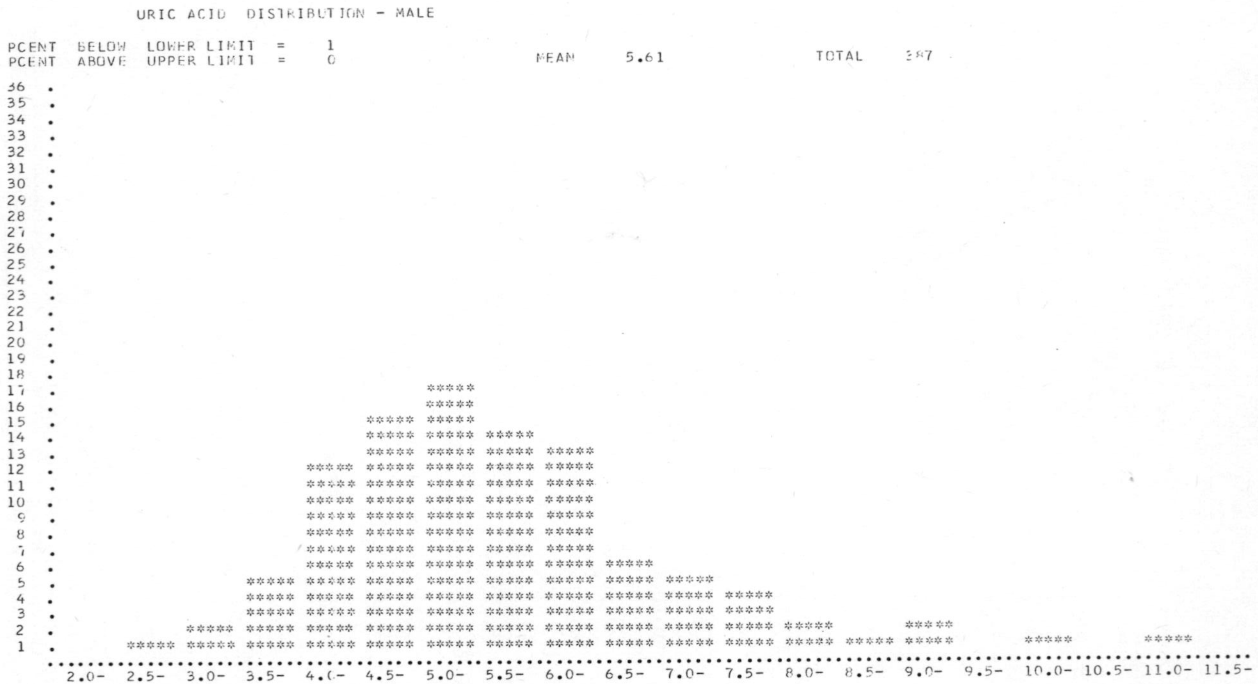

Fig. 9. Histogram showing the distribution of male uric acid results

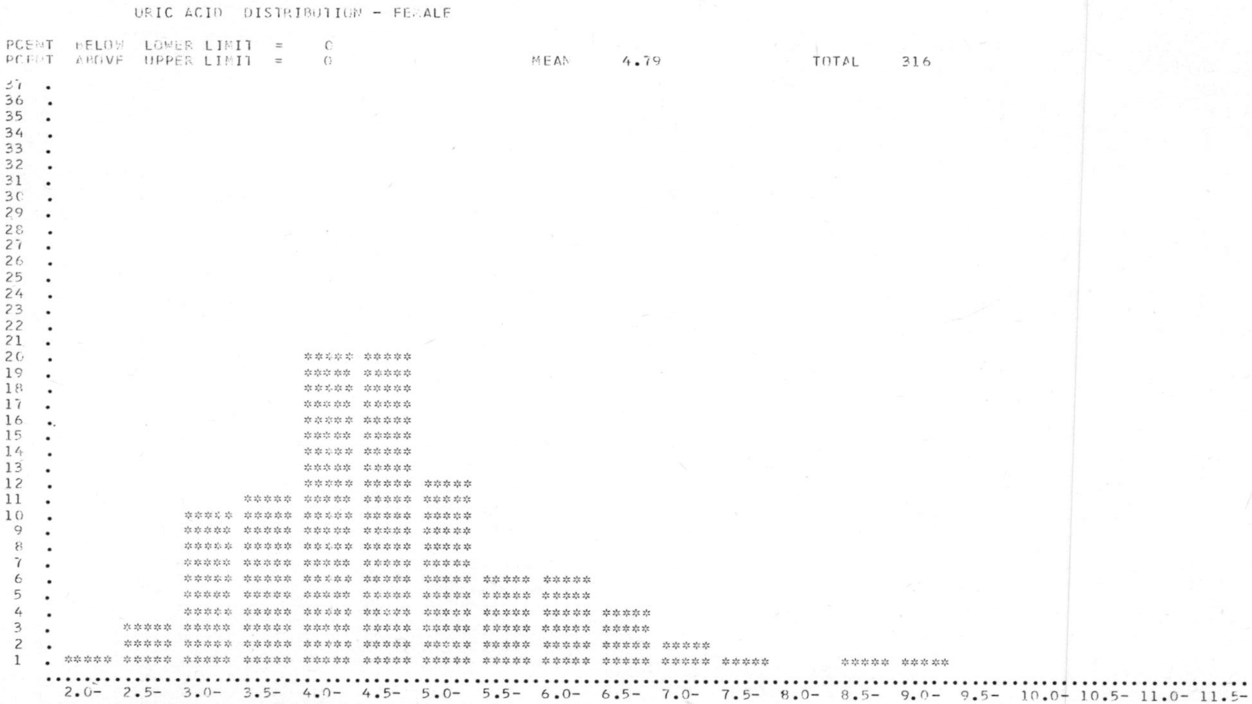

URIC ACID DISTRIBUTION - FEMALE

PCENT BELOW LOWER LIMIT = 0
PCENT ABOVE UPPER LIMIT = 0

MEAN 4.79   TOTAL 316

```
37 .
36 .
35 .
34 .
33 .
32 .
31 .
30 .
29 .
28 .
27 .
26 .
25 .
24 .
23 .
22 .
21 .
20 .                    *****  *****
19 .                    *****  *****
18 .                    *****  *****
17 .                    *****  *****
16 .                    *****  *****
15 .                    *****  *****
14 .                    *****  *****
13 .                    *****  *****
12 .                    *****  *****  *****
11 .             *****  *****  *****  *****
10 .             *****  *****  *****  *****
 9 .             *****  *****  *****  *****
 8 .             *****  *****  *****  *****                           *****
 7 .             *****  *****  *****  *****                    *****  *****
 6 .             *****  *****  *****  *****             *****  *****  *****
 5 .             *****  *****  *****  *****      *****  *****  *****  *****
 4 .      *****  *****  *****  *****  *****  *****  *****  *****  *****
 3 .      *****  *****  *****  *****  *****  *****  *****  *****  *****
 2 .      *****  *****  *****  *****  *****  *****  *****  *****  *****             *****  *****
 1 .      *****  *****  *****  *****  *****  *****  *****  *****  *****  *****  *****  *****  *****
    ................................................................................................................
    2.0- 2.5- 3.0- 3.5- 4.0- 4.5- 5.0- 5.5- 6.0- 6.5- 7.0- 7.5- 8.0- 8.5- 9.0- 9.5- 10.0- 10.5- 11.0- 11.5-
```

Fig. 10. Histogram showing the distribution of female uric acid results

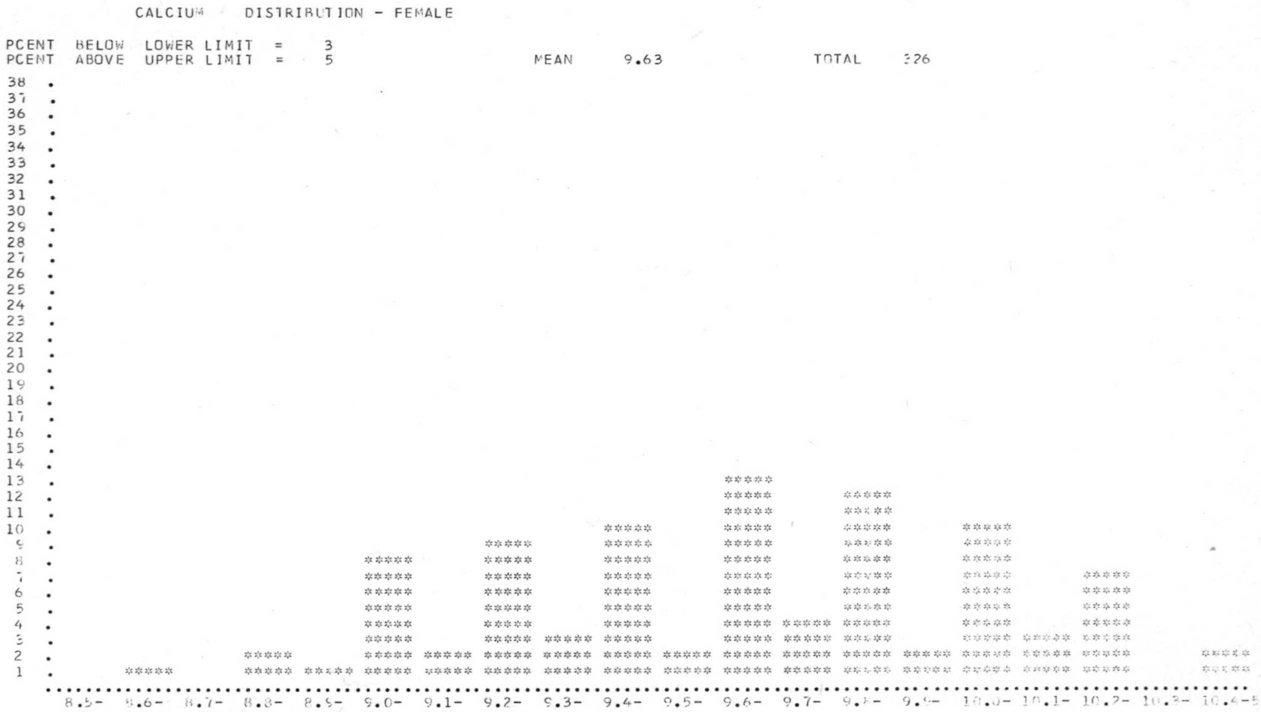

Fig. 11. Histogram obtained from an investigation of female serum calcium results

have values above the upper limit of normal whereas one in four males have values above 6.5 mg/100 ml.

Reading-off errors

Fig. 11 shows an interesting example of hidden data. It is evident from the distribution of results that technicians were biased against reporting numbers in the first place of decimals. Investigation showed that there was in fact a manual reading-off error which has now been corrected. Reading-off errors by technicians have been demonstrated in several methods and these were unknown prior to the use of the computer in handling data. In cumulative sum techniques a sustained change in slope of a cumulative sum graph indicates a consistent change in mean results. Fig. 12 shows a graph of the cumulative sum of mean urea values; it will be seen that the slope of the graph changed on several occasions during the period studied, the changes in slope corresponded to changes in technicians reading the results from an auto-analyser. Each technician had a positive or negative subjective bias in drawing the standard graph and reading off the results.

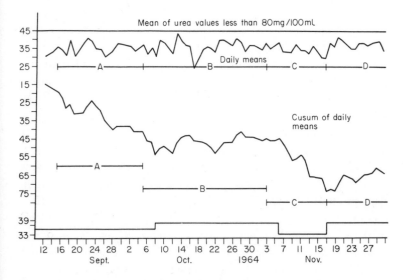

Fig. 12. Cumulative sum plot of daily means for serum urea

Cumulative reporting

There is one additional computer problem on which we have started work and this is the problem of handling results on file by the computer. The relationship of the most recent result from a particular patient with previous results on that patient is of importance to both the laboratory worker and the clinician in the ward. Thus, the preparation of a cumulative report containing all recent results is being actively studied at the present time. We are anxious to know the limitations and advantages of such techniques in laboratory management and patient care. There is increasing evidence that consideration of a series of results from one patient by 'thumbing through' a number of individual reports often leads to false impressions or a failure to notice important trends in results. When handling patients' results on computer files it is vital that patient identification should be always correct and it is for this reason that we have concentrated on communicating patient identification information in a machine-readable form.

DISCUSSION

The technique of data processing within the laboratory has achieved its first objective, that is, to reduce the clerical labour of the scientific staff in the laboratory and medical staff in the wards. In the laboratory the clerical labours of laboratory workers are now approximately 5 per cent of the total and this has been accomplished without increasing the clerical staff. Prior to the introduction of this system two clerks were used to prepare reports. Now a punch operator can deal in one day with approximately 250 requests equivalent to approximately 1000 tests. The average workload in the laboratory is under 200 specimens a day. At the same time the data produced by the laboratory is in a computer-readable form and this enables it to be used in the quality control and management of the laboratory. We now believe that efficient management in a laboratory as large as that in the Queen Elizabeth Hospital is only possible with the use of computer-orientated techniques.

In the use of the computer we have reached an important stage.

The programs which we routinely run on the IBM 1440 produce over 1000 figures each week and occasional programs such as the histogram program add further information all of which requires study and possible action. We have found the consideration of such data a formidable task and one that needs to be performed by senior staff. Many of the daily results can only be considered following the drawing of graphs. We have been successful in programing the computer to produce the points in a graph (Fig. 13), these points being joined by hand. This is a useful step, but an important development which is taking place at the present time is to program the computer to alert the laboratory staff to significant changes in control states. This is not only a more sophisticated programing problem but also a challenging situation to laboratory staff because they have to clearly state the situations about which they wish to be alerted. When such programs are available and in routine use we feel that we will be making proper use of the computer.

There remains one area of data handling in the laboratory which we have not yet been able to perform routinely on the computer, that is, the acquisition and calculation of a result. A study of this problem in this country and abroad has led us to conclude that this area of laboratory work requires the small scientific laboratory computer actually within the laboratory and on-line to the appropriate analytical instruments. Some of the laboratory management techniques mentioned above could also be performed at frequent intervals during the day. However, how far the small computer can be used for such techniques as well as acquiring analytical data could only be deduced from actual operating experience. We feel that the backing of a larger hospital computer will be essential for file handling and some laboratory management requirements. The off-line communication between the laboratory and the central hospital computer will also be the continuing subject of investigation.

We have only just begun to effectively use the data produced in the biochemistry laboratories in this hospital. Similar data-processing schemes to that outlined above are to be introduced in the other laboratories and this should enable us to link various

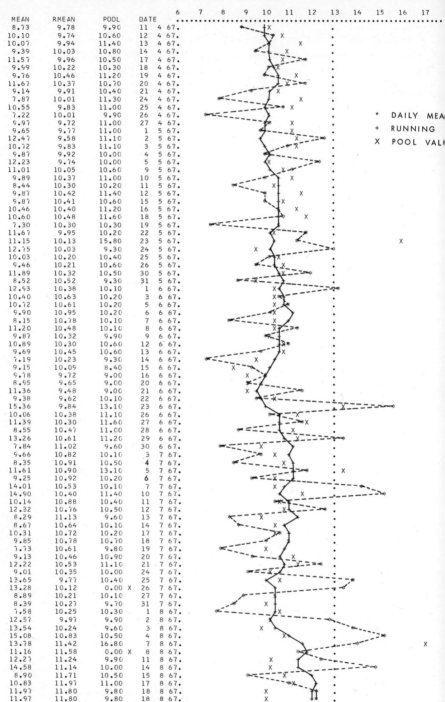

Fig. 13. Computer generated graph: the points of the graph have been manually connected

laboratory results on individual patients. We believe that the linking of data in this way could be even more fruitful than that realized in the biochemistry laboratory. Linking of clinical information with laboratory results is also an area of investigation which will be possible in the near future.

Acknowledgements

This work was made possible by research grants from the Medical Research Council, the Ministry of Health, the Endowment Fund of the United Birmingham Hospitals, and the Nuffield Provincial Hospitals Trust.

9

Radiotherapy treatment planning

R. F. FARR
J. A. NEWELL

*A small computer to hand is better than a
large one at a distance*

R. F. Farr, M.A., F.Inst.P., Hon.F.S.R.
Chief Physicist, United Birmingham Hospitals

J. A. Newell, M.A., D.Phil.
Principal Physicist, United Birmingham Hospitals

Radiotherapy treatment planning

The uniqueness of the individual patient

Radiotherapy treatment planning refers to the planning in respect of each individual patient of the manner in which the treatment shall be carried out to the best effect. It is a team effort involving radiotherapists, medical physicists, physics technicians, and radiographers. It is initiated by decisions on the part of the radiotherapist in respect of diagnosis, tumour location, and treatment policy. The end product is information and instructions which enable the radiographer to reproduce the prescribed treatment accurately, each day, over a period of weeks. Planning entails the use of various mechanical and electronic devices and involves extensive arithmetical calculations, most of which are best done with a computer.

The therapy as technique

Much of modern radiotherapy employs external beams of megavoltage radiation, for example, gamma rays from intense sources of cobalt-60 or 6–MV X-rays from linear accelerators. A particular feature of modern apparatus is its precise mechanical engineering which allows the axis of the beam to be directed accurately in space. In particular, however the beam is orientated, its axis passes through a single point in space, called the isocentre, with an accuracy of ± 2 mm.

The biological effect of such radiation is determined by *inter alia* the concentration of energy it delivers to tissue. This quantity is called the dose and the unit in which it is measured is the rad.

The tumour may be several centimetres beneath the surface of

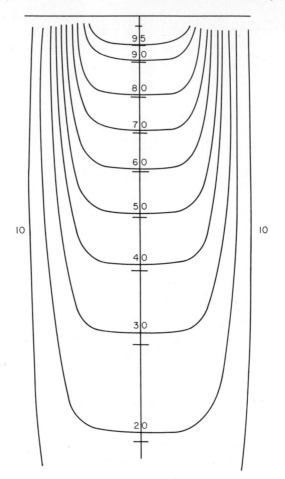

Fig. 1. A typical isodose chart used for manual computations

the body and the dose delivered at any depth is determined by the
thickness and nature of the intervening tissue. Basic measurements
with any given high energy beam are made in a phantom of water
(which well represents soft tissues), the beam being incident
perpendicularly upon a plane surface at a given distance from the
source. These data are usually expressed as isodose curves, i.e. a
family of lines joining points of equal relative dose (see Fig. 1). It
will be noted that the point of maximum dose (referred to as 100)

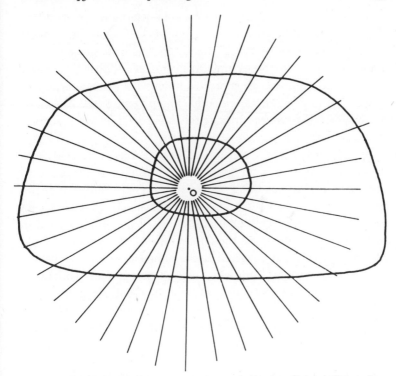

Fig. 2. Representation of body contour and tumour outline by radial co-ordinates along successive radii at 10° intervals

lies a few millimetres beneath the surface. (In fact, the computer has been used to calculate these curves from relatively limited experimental data thus reducing the amount of time for which access to the treatment machine is needed for such measurements.) For purposes of computation these data are expressed in digital form at intervals of 1 cm along radial lines at 10° intervals about the isocentre. Theoretical relations and the necessary data are available for correcting these data to the practical case where the beam is incident obliquely, the body surface is undulating and the source distance varies. These corrections are included in the computer program. Other corrections, for the effect of air space and bone, are usually applied *post hoc* as an empirical lump-sum correction.

A preliminary step is to determine the contour of the body

section in the region of the tumour and to determine the boundary of the volume to be treated in relation to it. Various mechanical aids and simulators are available and can be adapted to give their output in a form suitable as input to a computer. The body contour and tumour outline can be expressed in terms of polar co-ordinates about an arbitrary but conveniently chosen point o (see Fig. 2). It is convenient to measure and state the radial co-ordinates at angular intervals of 10°.

Since a single beam of radiation delivers a much smaller dose to the tumour than to innocent overlying tissue, it is necessary to employ more than one beam. These are directed at different angles and where they overlap their effects summate. In stationary field therapy, two, three, or four beams are used in turn, arranged in such a way as to minimize the dose received by innocent tissue in comparison with that delivered to the tumour.

In rotation therapy, with which this chapter is more particularly concerned, the beam rotates continuously about the isocentre so that, in effect, an infinite number of beams are applied in succession. For the purpose of computation it is regarded as occupying, successively, fixed directions at 10° intervals.

The calculation problems and the accuracy required

The beam may rotate through the full 360° or it may be switched off over selected arcs, to reduce the dose to particular organs or tissues. The object of the treatment plan is to choose the size of the beam, the location of the isocentre relative to the tumour, and any blank arcs, in such a way as to produce as uniform as possible a dose through the treated volume and as small as possible a dose to innocent tissue elsewhere. It will be affected by the size and location of the tumour and the patient outline and treatment plans are prepared in respect of individual patients.

The first choice of treatment parameters depends upon the judgement and experience of the planner. The resulting dose may be calculated at a number of points within the body—how many will depend upon the computing facilities and time available. Thus an hour or so spent at an electric desk calculator will provide the answer for 5–10 significant points in the body. This is clearly insufficient for a full evaluation of the treatment plan in respect of the individual patient. The first advantage of the computer is that it greatly increases the amount of data, the number of points at which the treatment dose is known, available to the clinician.

In the light of these results, the planner may decide to alter the basic treatment parameters to obtain a more favourable dose distribution. It is then necessary to repeat the whole calculation. The second advantage of the computer is therefore that it is able to produce for each patient a number of plans from which the most appropriate can be selected. In principle, this process of 'optimisation' can be carried out by the computer itself, if it can be given the criteria with which the choice should be made.

A third advantage is that the computer can be programmed to draw the final dose distribution as isodose curves much more quickly than a person could interpolate them from numerical data.

The computer application

In many centres in the United States, and a few in this country, computer programs have been operating for some time to produce radiation dosage distributions for specified treatments on individual patients. However, they have mostly used large and fast machines, and those who have used small machines have confined themselves to fixed-field treatments using a few fields. Rotational treatment must be regarded digitally as a number of fixed field treatments, but the number used must be more than a few in order to approximate to true rotation. We have taken rotation as represented by fixed fields at $10°$ intervals, giving a maximum of thirty-six such fields.

With the advent of an IBM 1440 computer in the hospital we had to decide whether to attempt to use it for rotational treatment planning. The 1440 is a decimal machine with a memory organized in characters. It is a machine designed for commercial use, for the input, output, and manipulation of large quantities of alphanumeric data. It is not designed for fast computation. Although the core-cycle time is not long (11 μsec), one cycle is required for the retrieval of each decimal digit of a number from the memory, whereas in machines designed for computation the whole of the number is retrieved in one cycle. This obviously increases the computation time by several orders of magnitude quite apart from the fact that decimal arithmetic takes longer to perform than binary. So would the attempt be worthwhile?

For the user, the amount of computer time used is, in a sense, irrelevant. The important thing is the 'turn-round'. The user wants to be sure of getting results back a known and reasonable time after handing them in. It is much better to get results in a few hours from a computer that has taken an hour to do the job than results in two or three days from a computer that has taken a minute. So it is obviously worth the attempt to use a slower computer within the hospital rather than a faster computer outside, where one would have to take one's turn with large numbers of other users. There is also, of course, advantage in using a computer that is a part of the hospital system because it is orientated to hospital use.

We already had available a programme written in Mercury Autocode for a KDF9. The principle we used was the same, but the vastly smaller memory and the very much lower speed of the 1440 forced us into drastic alterations of detail. Because of limitations of speed we are able to produce a dosage distribution for a prescribed treatment specification, but not at present to introduce any form of optimization within the programme.

Details of calculation

The field information, as explained above, is expressed as the dose received at each point of a polar grid with units of 1 cm along each radius up to 10 cm, the radii being at 10° intervals. Thus each field is described by 361 numbers. (For symmetrical fields this can be reduced to 191.) The dose at each point is that received in a phantom with a plane surface 65 cm from the source. The origin of the polar grid is the isocentre, at 75 cm from the source.

The dose delivered to points in the body is determined also at the 361 points of a polar grid with origin the centre of rotation of the source, i.e. the isocentre. If the body surface were a plane situated 10 cm from the isocentre, the actual dose delivered to each point would be equal to the dose in the field information for that point. Since it is not, a correction must be applied for each point.

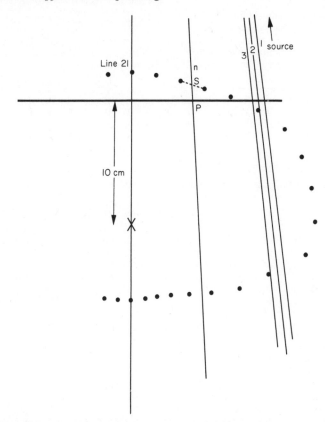

Fig. 3. Calculation of correction factor. The body contour is regarded as a series of straight lines joining adjacent points of the 36 that represent the contour. The intercept S, nearer the source, of line n with the body contour is determined. The distance d = SP is calculated. The correction factor for line n is then e $^{-\mu d}$ where μ is the absorption coefficient for the field used. The 41 correction factors are stored as calculated

This could be calculated for each of the 361 points. However, this would be time-consuming and unnecessary. We calculate for each source position, 41 possible correction factors, and then apply the most appropriate factor to each point in turn. This gives an error of no more than ±1 per cent compared with using 361 exact correction factors. Fig. 3 illustrates how the correction factor is obtained. A table, stored as constant data, indicates which is the appropriate correction factor to apply for each of the 361 points.

Name   Fletcher G.
Field size   8 * 8
Co-ordinates of centre of rotation   1·00,   180·00
Co-ordinates of body contour points

12·00	12·00	12·20	12·70	13·65	14·70	15·80	16·80	17·60	17·90	18·60	19·00
18·65	18·00	15·10	13·30	12·20	11·60	11·40	11·60	12·10	13·10	14·80	17·50
18·80	19·20	19·00	29·05	17·70	16·80	15·70	14·70	13·85	13·10	12·50	12·20

Treatment positions—F signifies blind arc

1	2	3	4	5	6	7	8	9	10	11	12	13	14	15	16	17	18
T	T	T	T	T	T	T	T	T	T	T	T	T	T	T	F	F	F
19	20	21	22	23	24	25	26	27	28	29	30	31	32	33	34	35	36
F	F	F	T	T	T	T	T	T	T	T	T	T	T	T	T	T	T

Fig. 4(a)

Doses at points on polar grid radius 10 cm. At intervals of 1 cm and 10 degrees—values are relative to central dose of 1000

Distance along radius

Radius		1	2	3	4	5	6	7	8	9	10
	1	1010	1026	1037	1014	925	791	672	591	537	501
	2	1010	1026	1037	1014	923	788	670	591	539	505
	3	1010	1026	1035	1008	917	781	665	590	541	508
	4	1010	1024	1031	1003	907	773	658	586	539	506
	5	1009	1021	1025	995	897	765	652	581	534	501
	6	1009	1018	1021	989	891	759	647	578	530	495
	7	1006	1115	1016	983	887	758	647	573	523	488
	8	1004	1011	1010	979	884	758	644	568	515	476
	9	1003	1007	1004	974	882	758	642	561	505	467
	10	1001	1003	997	967	879	755	638	555	500	462
	11	999	999	991	960	870	748	633	552	496	458
	12	999	995	986	950	857	739	628	552	497	459
	13	996	993	981	940	843	720	618	550	501	466
	14	994	990	976	932	828	697	595	535	496	471
	15	996	987	973	927	815	674	567	506	467	443
	16	992	985	970	923	807	657	544	477	436	406
	17	992	985	970	921	806	650	523	442	392	354
	18	991	984	968	920	809	651	508	410	339	288
	19	991	983	968	921	810	653	506	391	305	235
	20	991	983	967	919	809	654	511	410	340	288
	21	991	983	967	918	807	654	528	446	394	356
	22	991	984	966	918	806	660	551	486	442	411
	23	992	984	971	923	811	674	572	514	476	451
	24	992	986	971	926	822	694	596	539	504	480
	25	994	988	975	932	834	712	613	548	502	469
	26	996	990	978	940	847	725	614	541	488	451
	27	996	994	983	948	857	732	614	528	471	430
	28	999	996	988	956	863	737	615	529	466	424
	29	1000	1001	995	961	865	738	617	532	473	430
	30	1001	1006	1001	965	869	740	625	549	497	462
	31	1004	1009	1006	972	873	743	636	568	523	489
	32	1006	1014	1013	979	881	750	644	577	529	495
	33	1006	1017	1020	987	891	760	649	578	530	498
	34	1009	1021	1025	997	903	770	654	580	533	500
	35	1009	1023	1031	1006	915	779	661	584	534	502
	36	1010	1026	1035	1012	922	787	667	587	535	501

Fig. 4(b)

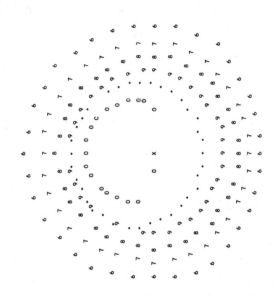

Fig. 4. (c)

Fig. 4. The three pages of computer output

(a). Patient information—name, field size, centre of rotation, body co-ordinates, treatment fields

(b). Tabular output—the normalized doses at points on a polar grid

(c). Contour output—pictorial representation of 4 (b) *Body outline . Tumour outline
  × Centre of rotation   0,9,8,7,6 100%, 90%, 80%, 70%, 60% of dose at ×

Initially, the dose at all the body points is set to zero. For the first source position, the actual dose at each body point is calculated as above and added to the dose already there, in this case zero. For the second source position, 10° from the first, the procedure is repeated. (We have, in fact, found it more convenient mathematically to rotate by 10° all the body co-ordinates, rather than the source position, as this then leaves the rest of the computation the same for each position.) Any positions, in which the beam is switched off, are omitted. The field specification points again overlie the body points and the correction factors are calculated and applied before adding the dose in. No interpolation is necessary. When the doses for all source positions have been added in, the doses are normalized with respect to 1000 at the isocentre, and the results printed out as a table (Fig. 4 (b)). It takes about fifty minutes to obtain this result.

The table gives accurate results but requires analysis to get a meaningful picture of dose distribution from it. When using a computer it is important that it should not leave much analysis still to be done, but that it should be made to complete the job and present a clear picture that can be immediately appreciated. We therefore use the results, that have been printed out as a table, to produce a contour map, to scale, of selected percentage doses. These are 100, 90, 80, 70, and 60 per cent of the dose at the iso-centre. Also printed out at the same time are the body contour points and the tumour outline so that the effectiveness of the treatment prescription can be visualized immediately. The line printer is an effective instrument for producing this output, which is obtained in about ten minutes. We do not consider that the use of a graph-plotter would give a significantly better output, and would probably increase the time for this part of the programme very considerably. Fig. 4 (c) shows a typical output. The tumour–air ratio printed at the top enables the actual dose delivered to be determined, and the patient's name is also printed for identification.

Input

The input to the program is the patient information and the appropriate field information. The latter is characteristic of the treatment machine and occupies ten punched cards per field size.

There are ten field sizes in current use. We have found it convenient to put all this field information on to magnetic tape and then to read the appropriate field information from the tape according to the field size specified on the patient card. The patient information is on eight punched cards. The first has the patient's name, field size, and co-ordinates of the centre of rotation. The next three have the body co-ordinates. The fifth contains information on the arcs to be omitted in treatment. The remaining three have the tumour co-ordinates. The program itself is stored on the magnetic disc which is an integral part of the computer system. All that is required for a run is two control cards, eight patient cards, a blank end-card, and the magnetic tape containing the field information. Any number of patients can be run consecutively with no intervention from the operator, a blank card indicating the end.

Considerations of time and storage

Careful attention needed to be given to time of execution. The original KDF9 program would have taken more than a day to run on the 1440. Time was saved by using forty-one correction factors instead of 361. Considerable time was also saved by realizing that some of the computation had already been done in previous computation. This may sound obvious but it is by no means always easy to discover. One general approach to the saving of time was governed by two rules—'Do not do what you do not have to' and 'Do not do again what you have already done.' The complete programme now takes just under one hour to run which is a manageable time on the hospital machine.

We have considered one hour to be about the maximum daily running time that a single department could reasonably expect to use on a computer installed for general hospital use. Had our machine been a fast one we should not have had to go to these lengths to reduce the time of execution. But in the circumstances we were forced to do so in order to gain the benefit of using the machine on the spot. This work will be of continued benefit even if a faster machine becomes available. It will then enable us to be much more elaborate and produce many alternative plans for one patient, and to do some form of computer-assisted optimization of treatment specification, while still keeping a reasonable total time. Without the constraint placed on us by a slow machine, we should be able to be much less elaborate on a fast machine within a given total execution time.

The constraint of small storage is another matter. This is nothing but a nuisance. A great deal of programming time is spent in arranging programs and variables to fit into a limited memory which need not be on a machine with larger memory. Furthermore, if a machine with larger memory becomes available, there will be no benefit at all to be gained from the work that has been done on account of small storage.

Summary

Computers are the obvious tool to use for radiotherapy treatment planning because of the large amount of calculation involved. This is particularly so for rotational treatment. Previously, these have usually been done on fast machines because of the length of the calculation. By careful pruning of the computations without sacrificing accuracy, we have been able to produce pictorial rotational plans on an IBM 1440, taking one hour per plan. It is very advantageous to be able to use this computer in the hospital itself rather than use a faster computer elsewhere. Furthermore, if a faster computer becomes available in the future, the saving in time that we have achieved in order to run the program at all on the 1440 will continue to be of benefit. We shall then be able to examine variations in plans and investigate methods of optimization to a much greater degree while keeping the running of the program within a reasonable total time.

Description of Program

PHASE 1 (INPUT)

Read from cards   Patient's name
(8 cards)   Field to be used   } (1).
                  Centre of rotation
                  Polar co-ordinates of body contour (2–4).
                  Source positions to be used (5).
                  Polar co-ordinates of tumour outline (6–8).

If first card is blank, stop.
Read from   Full specification of field named on first card.
magnetic tape

Print out (for identification) the information read from the cards.

Convert polar co-ordinates of contours to Cartesian co-ordinates with respect to centre of rotation.

Call Phase 2.

PHASE 2 (CALCULATION)

Initialize dose at all body points to zero.
Source position 1.
Check if treatment required at that source position.
If not, go to next position.
Calculate correction factors for each of 41 lines.

For each body point, take appropriate field data, multiply by appropriate correction factor and add result to dose already accumulated at that point.

Rotate body co-ordinates by 10°.

Repeat for next source position till all source positions used.

Print table of doses at all points of body on polar grid, normalized to 1000 at centre of rotation.

Call Phase 3.

PHASE 3 (CONTOUR OUTPUT)

Calculate 'tumour–air ratio' to give information on actual dose delivered at centre of rotation.

Print tumour–air ratio and patient's name.

Use doses calculated in previous Phase to find distances along each radius of 100, 90, 80, 70, and 60 per cent of dose at centre.

Convert these distances to X and Y positions on printing grid.

Convert body contour points and tumour outline in same way.

Print contour points, body points, and tumour points line by line with appropriate symbols.

Call Phase 1.

The computer and drug prescribing

O. L. WADE

Unexpected and exciting results

O. L. Wade, M.D., F.R.C.P.
Professor of Therapeutics and Pharmacology
The Queen's University of Belfast

The computer and drug prescribing

Northern Ireland has its own health service under which provision is made for the supply of drugs to patients who are under the care of their family doctor. As in England and Scotland prescriptions written by doctors on official forms (equivalent to the E.C. 10) are taken by the patients to pharmacists who supply the medicaments. The pharmacists retain the prescription forms and at the end of each month send them to the pricing bureau of the Northern Ireland General Health Services Board so that the cost of the drugs and service they have supplied can be paid.

In the early years of the Health Service the labour of examining and costing each prescription, which had to be done by specially trained staff, was so great that it was impossible to examine all the prescription forms and a one-in-ten sample of forms from each pharmacy was costed. This system of costing was found to lead to serious errors and sometimes caused hardship especially for small pharmacies from which only a few forms were received. In 1952 it was decided that all forms should be examined and costed. To do this the speed and efficiency of the pricing bureau was improved by the use of Hollerith punch cards with sorting and tabulating machinery, and the co-operation of all pharmacists was enlisted so that before they sent the forms to the pricing bureau they added to them code numbers indicating the particular pharmaceutical preparations and the quantities that they had supplied to the patients.

Shortly after the first reports of the thalidomide disaster (McBride, 1; Lenz, 2; Pfeiffer and Kosonow, 3), investigations of the incidence of amelia and other congenital deformities in relation to the prescribing of thalidomide in Scotland and Liverpool were hampered by the difficulties of tracing patients for whom the drug had been prescribed (Speirs, 4; Smithells, 5). The memory of women and the records of doctors about drugs which had been prescribed during pregnancy were unreliable. In the light of these reports the mechanized system used by the Northern Ireland General Health Services Board to cost prescriptions was examined. It seemed likely that with minor modifications it would be possible not only to characterize the prescribing of a particular drug by general practitioners but also to trace the names and addresses of every patient for whom it had been prescribed. This seemed so important in relation to the safe use of drugs in the community that an investigation of the prescribing of chloramphenicol was put in hand immediately (Wade, 6) in part to test the potentialities of the system and in part to investigate the relationship between the use of chloramphenicol and blood dyscrasias.

The chloramphenicol investigation

The following data for each item prescribed were routinely punched on the Hollerith cards:

> The code number of the pharmacy supplying the drug;
> The code number of the prescribing doctor;
> The code number of the pharmaceutical preparation prescribed;
> The code number of the quantity supplied;
> The script number: this allowed the original prescription form to be traced.

The cards for all prescriptions written during December 1962 were sorted and cards with the code numbers of preparations of chloramphenicol were extracted and analysed. In that month there were 3123 prescriptions for chloramphenicol. It was most frequently prescribed in the form of syrup, 1982 prescriptions, but the greatest quantity of chloramphenicol, 6100 G, was prescribed in the form of capsules for which there were 1141 prescriptions. The quantities supplied on each prescription were examined. The commonest quantity of syrup prescribed was 2 oz with a range of 1-8 oz. The most frequent number of capsules prescribed was 24 but between 12 and 60 capsules might be prescribed.

An analysis of the prescribing of individual doctors was made. There were 756 doctors in general practice in Northern Ireland at that time. Only 211 of them prescribed chloramphenicol syrup during that month. Most of the doctors wrote four or less prescriptions in the month but there were 24 doctors who wrote between 40 and 60 prescriptions and they prescribed more than half of the total amount of chloramphenicol syrup supplied in the month. Similarly only 243 doctors prescribed chloramphenicol capsules and the 30 doctors who wrote more than 10 prescriptions in the month prescribed more than one quarter of the total quantity of 6100 G supplied during the month. A further analysis of the prescribing of chloramphenicol in February 1964 suggested that there was persistence of the prescribing habit of individual doctors. Those who had been the heavy prescribers in December 1962 were for the most part the heavy prescribers in February 1964.

The records of all patients registered in Northern Ireland as dying from aplastic anaemia over the period 1960–4 were examined. There was no evidence that deaths from aplastic anaemia were disproportionately frequent amongst patients of practices in which there were doctors who were frequent prescribers of chloramphenicol, but for a number of reasons it was impossible to regard this negative finding as conclusive.

Tracing patients

Because all prescription forms were numbered and this number was recorded on the Hollerith card, it was possible, although a slow and tedious task, to trace and draw the original prescription forms written by general practitioners. On these forms were the names and addresses of the patients. It was this facility which seemed particularly important to the Committee on Safety of Drugs when it was formed in June 1963 and arrangements were made for prescription forms to be retained for a period of at least two years.

Occasion arose to test the value of this in 1964 when reports of animal studies suggested that the use of long-acting sulphonamide drugs during pregnancy might cause deformities of the foetus.

Within a few days it was possible to trace the names and addresses of all women who had received long-acting drugs nine months previously. Letters were then sent to their general practitioners: there was no evidence that the babies of those who had been pregnant when they received the drugs had been deformed.

The use of the British National Formulary (BNF)

With precautions to ensure confidentiality a random sample of prescriptions written in an urban area during June 1965 and all the prescriptions written by two doctors in a rural town were traced (7). The two doctors were chosen because their practices were of the same size and seemed to serve a similar cross-section of the community. One doctor, however, had prescribing costs which had been persistently above the average for Northern Ireland for many years and the other had costs persistently lower than the average.

Every prescription was examined to determine whether it was for:

1. A preparation in the current edition of the BNF;
2. A proprietary preparation for which either an exact equivalent in the BNF could have been prescribed, or if this was not possible, for which a BNF preparation could have been substituted which would have had substantially similar effects for the patient;
3. A proprietary preparation for which there was no suitable equivalent nor alternative in the BNF.

The results are shown in Table 1. The analysis of the random sample of prescriptions suggested that the BNF could meet almost all the requirements of prescribers in general practice. If the BNF preparations had been used it was difficult to conceive that the patients would have suffered to any appreciable extent and there would have been a reduction of about one-third in the cost of prescribing. As this amounts to about £4.4 million per annum in Northern Ireland a substantial saving of about £1 million per annum might be achieved.

There was only a small difference in the proportion of BNF preparations prescribed by the doctor who had high prescribing

Table 1. *Assessment of prescriptions*

	General sample No.	Practice A No.	Practice B No.
Total forms	455	968	969
Total prescriptions	695	1558	1294
For preparations from the BNF	110 (16%)	195 (13%)	313 (24%)
For proprietary preparations judged to have alternative in BNF	526 (76%)	1265 (81%)	866 (67%)
For proprietary preparations judged to have no alternative in BNF	32 (5%)	36 (2%)	75 (6%)
For dressings and appliances	27 (4%)	62 (4%)	46 (4%)

From Wade and McDevitt (7)

costs, 13 per cent of preparations from the BNF, and the doctor with low prescribing costs, 24 per cent of preparations from the BNF. The major difference accounting for the substantial difference in cost of prescribing between the two practices seemed to be due to the quantities of drugs prescribed. Thus if the high-cost practitioner prescribed a simple analgesic '2 tablets S.O.S.' he frequently ordered that 100 tablets be supplied, and if he prescribed an antacid mixture he frequently ordered 32 oz. If large supplies are needed by many patients it might have been expected that there would be evidence of more frequent visits by patients to the doctor who prescribed the small quantities, but this did not seem to be the case. The reasons for these differences in prescribing habit would clearly be worth investigating more fully.

THE COMPUTER AND PRESCRIBING

In April 1966 the Hollerith system was abandoned and the data from prescription forms was handled by electronic data-processing equipment. The speed and versatility that this has brought to the

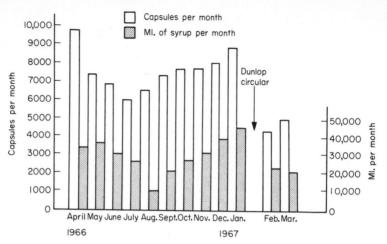

Fig. 1. The effect of a warning by the Committee on Safety of Drugs on the prescribing of chloramphenicol

analysis of prescribing has altered the range and scope of investigations that are now possible. All the work which was done slowly and tediously by sorting and tabulating Hollerith cards can now be done rapidly. What once took hours now takes minutes, and new and fascinating problems arise. One difficult challenge is to decide what portion of the torrent of available data should be examined. It is still too soon to give more than a brief account of some of the investigations which have been initiated with the help of a research assistant who was appointed in February 1967 with a grant from the Nuffield Provincial Hospitals Trust.

Factors which influence drug prescribing

Because it is now possible to get reliable data easily month by month on the prescribing of individual drugs it is possible to investigate factors which may influence prescribing. Fig. 1 shows changes in the amount of chloramphenicol prescribed which followed the warning about the hazards of the drug issued by the Committee on Safety of Drugs in January 1967.

The use of newly marketed preparations

There is little known of how individual doctors differ in their use

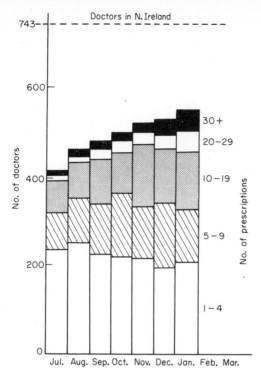

Fig. 2. Analysis of prescribing of a newly marketed hypnotic drug

of a newly marketed preparation. Fig. 2 shows one way in which this may be studied.

The geography of drug use

Because it is possible for the computer to print out in a few moments details of the prescribing of a particular drug by every practitioner in Northern Ireland, it is possible to construct maps showing the use of drugs in the community. One of the first studies has shown that the use of insulin is remarkably uniform throughout Northern Ireland, but there are remarkable differences in the prescribing of oral anti-diabetic drugs (Fig. 3). In some urban areas in the south-east, for instance, these drugs are widely prescribed and in similar areas in the north-west they are infrequently prescribed. The prescribing of thyroid, thyroxine, and antithyroid

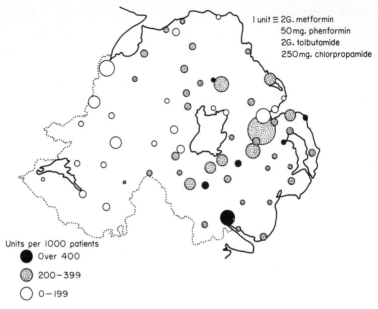

I unit ≡ 2G. metformin
50 mg. phenformin
2G. tolbutamide
250 mg. chlorpropamide

Units per 1000 patients
● Over 400
⊛ 200–399
○ 0–199

Fig. 3. The prescribing of oral antidiabetic drugs in Northern Ireland in January 1967.

drugs also varies greatly. They all seem to be highly prescribed along the sea coast and around Lough Neagh. Interpretation of these findings is going to require further investigation but already new, fascinating, and unexpected ideas are arising.

CONCLUSIONS

Two features of this work have given special satisfaction. First there has been the delight of the unexpected. In 1962 the problem was to devise a method of tracing all patients who had received a particular drug. This has led to unpredicted and unpredictable forms of operational research which are only possible because electronic data-processing equipment has been developed and is accessible. This operational research is now presenting a profusion of novel, difficult and disturbing ideas and concepts.

Secondly, there has been the satisfaction of showing that such a mundane procedure as the costing of prescriptions can be used to reveal useful insight about disease, patients, and doctors. This is the satisfaction of the cook who finds old left-overs in the kitchen and creates a splendid dish. The more unpromising the initial ingredients the greater the sense of achievement.

Acknowledgements

By the nature of this work I have had many helpers. I am indebted to colleagues in my Department and in particular to Mrs. Helen Hood, Dr. D. G. McDevitt, and Professor P. C. Elmes. I acknowledge that these studies have been made possible by the wholehearted co-operation I have received throughout from Mr. A. W. Kernahan, Pharmaceutical Officer to the Northern Ireland General Health Services Board and the staff of the Pricing Bureau. I am deeply indebted to Mr. G. D. Stewart, Secretary of the Board and Dr. R. P. Maybin, Medical Officer of the Board. I would like to thank Dr. F. Main, Chief Medical Officer, and the many officers in the Northern Ireland Ministry of Health and the Government Computer Services who have so readily given help and encouragement. I gratefully acknowledge the grant made by the Nuffield Provincial Hospitals Trust in support of these studies.

References

1. McBride, W. G. (1961). *Lancet*, ii, 1358.
2. Lenz, W. (1962). Ibid., i, 45.
3. Pfeiffer, R. A., and Kosenow, W. (1962). Ibid. i, 45.
4. Speirs, A. L. (1962). Ibid. i, 303-5.
5. Smithells, R. W. (1962). Ibid. i, 1270-3.
6. Wade, O. L. (1966). *J. Coll. Gen. Practit.* 12, 277-86.
7. —— and McDevitt, D. G. (1966). *Brit. Med. J.* 2, 635-7.

11

The development of drug monitoring for side-effects within a hospital medical information system

R. D. WEIR
J. CROOKS
D. C. COULL

Recording side-effects has raised many wider issues

R. D. Weir, M.D., D.P.H.

Senior Lecturer
Department of Public Health and Social Medicine
University of Aberdeen

J. Crooks, M.D., F.R.C.P. (Ed.&G.)

Reader in Therapeutics and Pharmacology
University of Aberdeen

Dorothy C. Coull, M.B., Ch.B.

Ciba Research Fellow
Department of Therapeutics and Pharmacology
University of Aberdeen

The development of drug monitoring for side-effects within a hospital medical information system

The vast number of pharmacologically active and therapeutically effective drugs which have become available in the last two decades has produced a revolution in the practice of medicine. It was, of course, realized that the price of these remarkable therapeutic advances was being paid in an increased frequency of unwanted side-effects but this realization did not produce a serious attempt to tackle this problem until the thalidomide disaster and with this event the absolute necessity of monitoring drugs for side-effects was accepted both at a medical and a political level.

The first attempts to obtain the information on which an adequate system of drug monitoring must be based has highlighted the world-wide inadequacy of medical information systems both in respect of the recording and collection of such data (1). Thus many of the problems discussed in this paper are as applicable to the handling of medical information in general as they are to drug monitoring.

As in any field of scientific investigation it is naive to believe that the problems of drug monitoring can be tackled without first investigating methodology, i.e. the techniques of recording, collecting, and evaluating data, and this description of the work carried out in Aberdeen and its potential developments concentrates on this approach.

Drug monitoring has two major objectives:

(i) To establish the frequency of side-effects both well recognized or newly discovered; and

(ii) To detect unexpected side-effects.

To successfully achieve the first objective requires a complete record of all prescriptions of a drug suspected of producing a well recognized side-effect or a newly identified one in the individuals from a total population who have received that drug and who therefore are at risk. The second objective can only be achieved by recording all events which happen to patients together with the drugs they are taking at the time of the event. Some of these events can be explained on the basis of the disease from which the patient suffers and others by recognized side-effects of the drugs he is taking. The unexplained events are thus potentially due to unrecognized effects of these drugs (2).

The collection of information of the above type is not easy; because a drug has been prescribed it does not necessarily follow that the drug has in fact been administered or that the dosage is correct. Prescriptions are frequently in a form that allow neither easy recognition nor recording and the sheer volume of prescribing creates, in itself, a formidable difficulty. The ascertainment of unexplained events also presents great difficulties even when they are manifest by the development of obvious signs and symptoms since it cannot be assumed that when they are observed these are always reported and recorded (3). The position is further complicated by the fact that patients frequently receive a number of drugs at the same time and allowance must be made for the possibility that one or a combination of two or more may be responsible for the event. For example, in the medical units of Aberdeen Royal Infirmary patients, on average, receive more than four drugs during their period of admission and 20 per cent of them receive more than ten drugs (4). Furthermore, account must be taken of the possible effects of drugs in relation to different pathological conditions from which the patients are suffering and which may not necessarily be the disease under treatment.

The methodological problems that must be resolved to obtain meaningful data in a drug monitoring system are thus:

a. The development of a standard and clear form of prescribing;

b. A method of checking the actual administration of drugs;

    c. The linkage of all drugs prescribed for individual patients together with the related diagnoses;

    d. The ascertainment of events happening to the patients, both explained and unexplained using a procedure which will allow comparison of the relative accuracy of the various sources providing such information.

    e. Because of the volume of this information, the development of computer techniques for its handling, storage, and analysis.

One of the major features stimulating the development of a scheme for drug monitoring in the north-east of Scotland was the introduction of a standard form of hospital prescribing (5). This has made possible the production on machine punch cards, of a complete index of all drugs prescribed within any of the units or hospitals in the area. While the accumulation of this information is an essential prerequisite for drug monitoring it is also possible to use the drug index for other purposes such as the comparative analyses of prescribing patterns with time (6).

Associated with the development of the new prescribing system was a method of recording the actual administration of individual drugs (7) and while originally devised as part of the monitoring programme these records are now also routinely analysed to provide the senior nurses with comparative measures of performance in patient management.

Drug records pertaining to individual patients are also linked by means of punch cards, to diagnoses and other information concerning an admission or hospital attendance. Plans are presently being prepared to extend this type of data linkage on a regional basis (8), into which at a later stage it may be possible to introduce data from domiciliary practice. As a result of this, information concerning patients, the diseases from which they are suffering, and the drugs which they have received is being collected for a series of complete and defined populations. By examination of hospital and domiciliary records and interviews with the patients the period and dosage of drug exposure could be related to the actual frequency of specified side-effects. Such a system could then be used by the

Committee on the Safety of Drugs to investigate reports made to the 'Early Warning Scheme'.

The information made available would also allow the subdivision of patients at risk by diagnosed pathological conditions and by concomitant exposure to various drug combinations. For this purpose computer facilities would be essential and a number of specific techniques to handle such data would be required. These include the creation of drug and diagnostic dictionaries and the development of alternative forms of recording to improve on conventional input techniques currently involving transcription, uneconomic in time and money.

The next stage is to relate these data to the potential side-effects of these drugs within the same groups of patients but the methodological problems involved are much more complex. Outside specific projects the recording of response to drugs is seldom made in a systematic fashion. In view of these difficulties a series of studies were undertaken in Aberdeen, in which over 1000 case records were examined, to evaluate the information that was available and to explore the possibility of designing new records or modifying existing ones for the purposes of monitoring. There appeared to be four possible sources of such information: first, the creation of a specially designed monitoring record; second, the existing medical progress notes; third, the daily nursing reports; and fourth, reports of laboratory tests. The analysis showed that although the creation of a special record initially provided excellent data the quality diminished with time (9); furthermore, marked differences were also found between the routine reports of medical and nursing staff. In general, medical reports tended to concentrate on major events such as blood dyscrasias, respiratory, and cardiovascular complications while the nursing notes included a far more extensive account of patients' activities and complaints.

An attempt was then made to estimate the extent to which the information actually recorded in the routine notes represented the total information that could reasonably have been obtained. For this purpose ninety-two patients were studied for a period of one month, after which three separate sources of data were compared. These sources were:

a. The results of daily interview with each patient by a doctor who although familiar with the ward was not on routine duties during the period;

b. The daily nursing reports; and

c. The corresponding medical progress notes.

It was assumed for the purposes of the study that the items obtained by interview represented the total information that could have been obtained. This appeared to be the only practical measure to use and as medical staff could never be employed for this purpose on a large scale it was felt that if the existing routine reports approximated to the interview data then it would be feasible to develop these sources for the purposes of monitoring. The events reported were then classified and compared. In this presentation an 'event' refers to a sign or symptom reported by the observer and an 'event day' indicates the number of occasions on which the 'event' could have been reported. (For example, if a patient had diarrhoea for four days this is reported as one 'event' and as four 'event days'.) A distinction is also made between events readily accounted for by the diagnosis and those not so explained. The majority of explicable 'events' were, in fact, recorded during the early days of a patient's admission (for example, chest pain with myocardial infarction or nausea and vomiting with duodenal ulceration). The results of the comparison are shown in Tables 1 and 2.

Although on five occasions the nurses reported 'events' omitted by the interviewing doctor, over-all, the nursing reports were found to include over 65 per cent and the medical progress notes less than 5 per cent of the possible total. For 'events' not readily explained by the diagnosis the proportions were 60 per cent for the nursing reports and 9 per cent for medical progress notes. From an examination of the 'event days' it appeared that the longer a symptom persisted the greater were the chances that it would be reported although there was some evidence to suggest that once a symptom had been recorded it was less likely to be reported on subsequent days. A detailed analysis which included the frequency with which

Table 1. *A comparison of 'events' recorded by special interview and routine ward reports for ninety-two patients over a period of thirty days*

Source of data	'Events' readily explained by the diagnosis	'Events' not explained by the diagnosis	Total number of 'events' reported
Interview schedule	44	177	221
Nursing report	46	103	149
Medical progress notes	27	17	44

Table 2. *A comparison of 'event days' recorded by special interview and routine ward reports for ninety-two patients over a period of thirty days*

Source of data	'Event days' explained by diagnosis	'Event days' not explained by diagnosis	Total number of 'event days' reported
Interview schedule	210	568	768
Nursing report	113	179	292
Medical progress notes	47	24	71

particular words and phrases were used showed that the omissions in the nursing reports were not associated with particular disease or symptom groups. The nursing reports, however, frequently omitted 'events' based on laboratory tests or the results of special examinations; however, a high proportion of the reporting by doctors dealt with major 'events'. An examination was also made of the laboratory investigations carried out on the same group of ninety-two patients. In all 1355 biochemical investigations were requested of which 292 produced results outside the accepted range of normality. Of these 292 'abnormal' results 177 (60 per cent) could not be explained solely by the diagnoses made while in hospital. It is not suggested that all inexplicable laboratory results and symptoms are due to the effects of drugs but within this, as yet, unordered mass of figures and words there lie valuable data that could be used in drug monitoring.

Although these findings were not entirely unexpected they point the need to systematize the recording of medical, nursing and laboratory information. Once a system has been devised which will simplify both the recording and analysis of these data then it will be possible not only to improve the quality of the material collected but to assess its significance as an indicator of established, suspected or previously unrecognized drug reactions. Development of these methods would make a major contribution to the organization of medical information for systematic analysis. With this facility possible associations between symptom complexes, laboratory findings, and specific drugs might be recognized and thus supplement the present method of detecting potential hazards by reports to the 'Early Warning Scheme'. Full exploitation of drug monitoring techniques would be dependent on a number of other developments which include advances in laboratory techniques and records, a complete change in the collection and recording of all types of medical information and the creation of a binary translator language to handle the vast amount of data that would be generated.

There is no quick or easy way of dealing with these problems, but given adequate facilities, the application of computer techniques point the way to a solution. Urgent though the problem of drug monitoring is, the cost and labour involved in an ideal system could not be contemplated unless it was closely linked to other applications of a composite medical information system. As many of the other articles in this publication show, a proportion of the techniques needed for such systems have already been established. Indeed, the investigation of methods for the detection and control of adverse drug reactions might well provide an added stimulus to the further development and application of medical information systems which if successful would transform medical practice in the future.

References

1. World Health Organisation (1965). *Report by the Director General to the 37th Session on International Monitoring of adverse reactions to drugs.*
2. FINNEY, D. J. (1965). *J. Chron. Dis.* 18, 77.
3. LASAGNA, L. (1964). *Prospect. Biol. Med.* 7, 4, 457.

4. Pharmaceutical Services Committee—Aberdeen General Hospitals (1966–7). Information Bulletins.

5. CROOKS, J., CLARK, C. G., CAIE, H. B., and MANSON, W. B. (1965). *Lancet*, i, 373.

6. King's Fund Hospital Centre Conference Report (1967). *Drugs in Hospital*.

7. CROOKS, J., WEIR, R. D., COULL, D. C., MCNAB, J. W., CALDER, G., BARNETT, J. W., and CAIE, H. B. (1967). *Lancet*, i, 668.

8. Oxford Record Linkage Study International Symposium 1967, 'Record Linkage' (to be published).

9. COULL, D. C. (1967). Personal communication.

12

The Exeter Community Health Research Project

J. R. ASHFORD
N. G. PEARSON

Possibilities for a joint computer service in a community

J. R. Ashford, M.A., Ph.D.
Professor of Statistics
University of Exeter

N. G. Pearson, M.B., B.S.
Clinical Epidemiologist
Exeter Community Health Research Project
University of Exeter

The Exeter Community Health Research Project

1. Introduction

The Exeter Community Health Research Project is a long-term epidemiological study of health problems in the city of Exeter. The research has three main objectives: firstly, to demonstrate the total incidence of illness brought to medical attention among as large a section as possible of the population of the city of Exeter over a period of one year; secondly, to correlate morbidity experience with personal information; and thirdly, to investigate in depth specific problems brought to light by the morbidity survey, including the application of computers within the health services. The first stage of the research comprises a one-year morbidity survey. During this period a record is being made of all morbidity reported to general practitioners or to hospitals. To supplement this information about sickness, brief personal particulars obtained from the general practice lists have also been recorded. In addition, a private census dealing with personal factors in greater detail is being conducted.

The large quantities of information generated by the research are being processed and analysed using unit record machines in the University of Exeter and the IBM 7090 computer at Imperial College, London. Although this project is being undertaken solely with a view to epidemiological research, it is apparent that much of the information being recorded and processed has potentially an immediate application to both day-to-day and long-term conduct of the health services in Exeter. Furthermore, the methods already in operation for data collection and analysis have provided a practical

Table 1. *Exeter Community Health Study. Summary of information collected*

Type	Source	Remarks
Registration	General practice	Minimal personal information for each patient on general practice lists
Census	Special census of city of Exeter	More detailed personal information together with data about household
Consultation	General practice	Brief details of each confrontation between patient and general practitioners
Hospital	Local hospitals	Brief details of each out-patient consultation and each in-patient admission and/or discharge

demonstration of the application of computer techniques in the general field of community medicine.

2. Sources of basic information

The main sources of information used for the project are listed briefly at Table 1. The survey population is defined by the general practice lists of the 35 (out of 49) practitioners working in Exeter who have agreed to take part in the survey. Some 70 000 patients are involved, representing just over three-quarters of the population of about 90 000 of the city of Exeter. The morbidity survey is confined to NHS patients only and the very small proportion of private patients has been excluded from the study. Although the general practices included in the survey are self-selected by virtue of the willingness of the doctors concerned to participate, it appears that the survey population is reasonably representative of the whole city.

a. Registration. For convenience of data processing each patient is identified by a special six-digit number, the first two digits corresponding to a code for the general practice involved. The first stage of the survey was the registration of the patients, which was carried out by reference to the NHS records kept by the general practitioners. A set of self-adhesive numbers, preprinted in triplicate, was used as a basis for the identification of patient records. The first number was used to identify the NHS envelope kept in the general practice, the second to identify the special consultation record card (see below) used for the survey (which was placed within each envelope) and the third was used as part of a manuscript register kept in alphabetical order of surname showing the name, identification number, date of birth, and address of each patient registered with the practice. The name and address of the patient was also noted on the consultation record card.

Not unexpectedly, it was found during the course of the registration operation that many of the general practice records were incomplete. Addresses were often many years out of date and information about the age of the patient was frequently either missing altogether or inaccurate. Furthermore, a proportion of the records referred to patients who had left the district or were dead. The registration process was carried out during the summer of 1966 with the help of a team of students. Changes in the composition of the participating general practices taking place subsequently are notified as they occur, using the same system as for the original registration.

b. Census. In view of the lack of reliable data about the personal characteristics of the patients available from the general practice records it was considered necessary to carry out a special inquiry in an attempt to obtain further information. Following a pilot study in the autumn of 1966, a private census was undertaken during the summer of 1967. This census was based on up-to-date rating valuation lists provided by the Exeter City Council, which show both address and rateable value. The whole of the city of Exeter was covered, including households and individuals whose general practitioner was not taking part in the morbidity survey. A trained interviewer visited each address on this list and put a standard series of questions to a responsible member of the household concerned. The inquiry is divided into two parts, the first being concerned with the household itself and the second with the individuals living in the household. Information collected about the household includes rateable value, occupation, industry, and employment status of the head of the household, and details of the type of living accommodation and amenities available. Both the latter sets of information were collected in a comparable way to that used by the General Register Office on their 1966 one-in-ten census of England and Wales. Details were also recorded about domestic pets. For each individual living in the household information was obtained about date and place of birth, residential history, marital status, educational standard, and family size, together with a record of smoking habits compiled by using the same form of enquiry as that recommended by the MRC Committee on the Aetiology of Chronic Bronchitis (MRC, 1).

c. **General practice consultations.** As part of the initial registration operation a manuscript record card (Fig. 1) was inserted in the NHS envelope for each patient on the general practice lists. This document makes provision for recording each professional confrontation between doctor and patient either at home, in the surgery, or elsewhere. Corresponding to every such event an entry is made by the general practitioner showing the day and month of the consultation, the diagnosis or principal symptom, the place of the consultation, a code corresponding to items of certification, and whether or not the patient was referred to a hospital or elsewhere. Allowance is made for consultations involving multiple diagnoses or symptoms, in which case a separate entry is made for each such diagnosis or symptom. The consultations are numbered serially throughout the survey year and the diagnoses are numbered serially within each consultation. Provision is also made for correcting previous diagnoses in the light of any information which subsequently becomes available, a separate entry being made for the correction to each incorrect diagnosis. It was originally intended to record telephone contacts between doctor and patient, but a pilot study showed that this was impracticable and a record of telephone activities is being made, on a sample basis only, at selected practices and for limited periods. Following a series of short pilot studies the main morbidity study began at the beginning of October 1966,

**EXETER GENERAL
PRACTICE MORBIDITY
SURVEY**

Surname	Forenames
....	....

Address ....

Date of Birth..

1	2
3	4

Date	Cons. No.	Diag. No.	Diagnosis	Corr.	Cert.	In.	Pl./ Tel.

REFERRAL No.	Where referred

DPS (T/3952)

Fig 1. Example of record card used by the General Practitioner to record morbidity

and continued until November 1967. All the General Practitioners taking part were able to complete the standard consultation records throughout the whole twelve months of the survey.

d. Hospital records. At each of the forty-four hospitals and nursing homes in the Exeter area a record is being made of all out-patient consultations and in-patient admissions and discharges of patients belonging to the defined population. The hospital out-patient records are similar in general form to the general practice consultation records. Each consultant or other member of the medical staff conducting an out-patient clinic makes a special record showing his diagnosis or the principal symptom involved on a small slip which is attached to the patient's notes. Arrangements have been made with the general practitioners and with the hospital records staff to include the patient identification number on all patient records used by the hospital including this special record. The hospital admission and discharge registers are used to provide information about in-patients coming from the defined general practices. A separate record is made of each admission and discharge, showing the date, the principal diagnosis, the hospital, the specialty, and the consultant concerned. This information has been collected since the beginning of the morbidity survey in October 1966 and the total of fifty-seven consultants concerned have provided a full cover of all the morbidity reaching the local hospitals throughout the survey year.

3. Data collection and processing
In view of the large quantities of information collected and the disparate sources involved it was decided to use mark sense punch cards as the basic medium for recording the data. Examples of all the cards used in the research are shown at Figs. 1–4. These cards are easily transportable and the information is recorded in pre-coded form by making pencil marks in the appropriate boxes on the card. The mark sense cards are then processed by a special machine and holes are punched in the cards corresponding to the pencil marks. Because of the amount of information collected, both

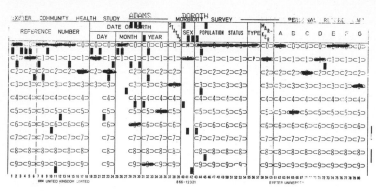

Fig. 2. Example of mark sense card used for registration of patients

the household and the personal records used on the census are printed and marked on both sides.

a. Registration. During the course of the registration operation a mark sense card was made out for each patient, showing reference number, date of birth, address (coded in terms of seven digits) and other factors as shown in Fig. 2. The name of the patient is also written (in ink) on the card. After mark sense punching, the name was hand-punched into the card. In order to deal with patients who join or leave the practice during the course of the survey year, a special code is entered in the columns assigned to 'population status'.

b. Census. The two cards used in the census are shown at Fig. 3. Most of the information collected was mark-sensed during the course of the interview, although name, occupation, industry and employment status were entered in manuscript. Certain items, including rateable value, social class, socio-economic group, and type of occupation were coded and mark sensed at a later stage. The reference number corresponding to each personal card was identified by consulting the manuscript register prepared as part of the registration operation. Patients registered with general practitioners not participating in the survey or patients not registered with any doctor were assigned numbers from a special series.

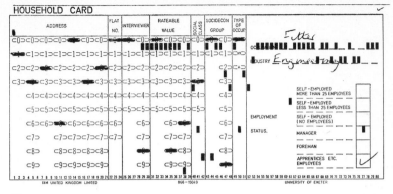

Front

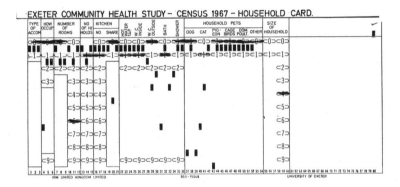

Back

Fig. 3. Example of mark sense card used for the private census *a*. Household card

c. General practice consultations.

Reference to Fig. 4 shows that the information collected on the consultation mark sense card agrees very closely with the doctor's manuscript record. Each record card corresponds to a line of the general practitioner's manuscript. The reference number is that given on the preprinted label, and the date, consultation number, and diagnosis number are as recorded by the doctor. The diagnosis or principal symptom noted in plain language by the doctor (see Fig. 1) is coded in accordance with the International Classification of Diseases (WHO,

PERSONAL CARD

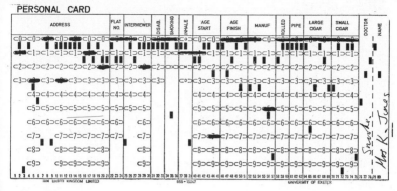

Front

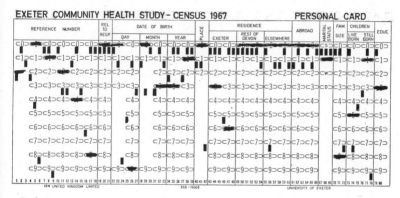

Back

Fig. 3 *b*. Personal card

2). Separate codes have been evolved to deal with items of certification, with the initials of the doctor concerned and with referrals. Apart from pilot trials which were carried out to prove the practicability of the system, the processing of information from the manuscript records was deferred until the end of the morbidity survey year in November 1967. At this stage the name and address of the patients are obscured before the cards are coded by specially trained medical auxiliaries. In this way the confidentiality of the morbidity information is preserved.

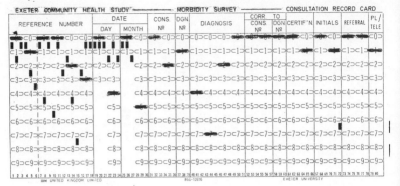

Example of mark sense card used for general practice records

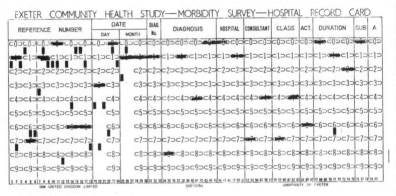

Example of mark sense card used for hospital records

Fig. 4

d. Hospital records. The same hospital record card is used both for out-patient appointments and also for in-patient admissions and discharges, as shown in Fig. 4. As with the general practice consultation records, the diagnosis or symptom is coded in accordance with the International Classification of Diseases. Separate codes are used for the hospital, the consultant, the type of specialty, and the action resulting from the event recorded. The columns assigned to duration on this card are used only in the case of hospital discharges, when they refer to length of stay in the hospital.

e. Data handling. A uniform method of processing and recording is used for each source of data. When the appropriate punch cards from a given source have been run through the mark sense punch they are sorted into identification number order. The cards are then taken to the IBM 7090 computer at Imperial College and are written on to magnetic tape. This operation is basically a process of updating magnetic tape files and all the computer programmes concerned have the same general structure. Whilst this operation is being carried out the computer checks on the internal consistency and validity of the new records and, where appropriate, also assesses the validity of the patient's composite record including 'new' and 'old' information. As a result, a set of magnetic tape files corresponding to each of the four basic sources of information is maintained, in every case the information being stored in identification number order.

4. Record linkage and analysis

Since all items of information are identified by means of a single number, the linkage of data from several sources is a comparatively straightforward undertaking. When two or more sources of data are to be linked, the magnetic tapes concerned are coupled to different tape readers on the computer. The two or more tapes are then read simultaneously by the machine and information from the different sources corresponding to the same reference number is brought together.

The analysis of the data collected falls into two main parts. First is the assessment of each source of information separately. When this is done the single tape concerned is loaded on to a tape unit and by means of a suitable programme any necessary computations are carried out on the basis of the data of this tape. For example, an age/sex register of a given general practice population may be obtained by a simple analysis of the tape containing the registration information. Similarly, a study of the work-load of a given hospital consultant may be obtained by an analysis of the hospital record tape.

Secondly, more complex analyses involving multiple sources of information may be carried out by loading several tapes at the same time. For example, if a study is to be made of the relation between household data and a particular type of illness, the general practice consultation record and census tapes may be analysed simultaneously. The IBM 7090 computer (which was replaced by the more modern 7094 machine in March 1968) is capable of dealing with input from as many as eight tape units simultaneously. This facility makes it possible to carry out very complicated statistical analyses as required.

5. Discussion

The successful completion of the morbidity survey in November 1967 has provided a practical confirmation of the basic methodology used for the collection and handling of the data. In the first place, a standard method of recording sickness in a large community as it occurs has been established. The procedures used have been shown to work efficiently for both general practice and hospital records and could be extended with very little difficulty to the local authority fields. Secondly, a record linkage operation bringing together data from various sources has been achieved. In this way it is possible to produce an integrated patient record. Thirdly, the general systems and procedures have proved capable of dealing with a group of some 70 000 individual patients and their extension to populations of as large as, say, 500 000 would involve no new principles. In general, an information system has been established which could be adapted and extended to provide a useful service in the community.

As far as the techniques of data collection and analysis are concerned, the basic method of recording by the use of mark sense cards has proved satisfactory over a wide variety of conditions. Up to the present time more than 100 people of varying degrees of skill and experience have recorded information in this form with uniform success. The full potential of the method was realized on the private census when two-sided punch cards were mark sensed 'on the doorstep'. By the use of this technique great savings of time and cost are being achieved in comparison with alternative methods such as the punching of cards from manuscript documents. The next step of the programme of data processing involves the transfer of information from the punch cards to a magnetic medium for computer analysis. This operation is greatly handicapped by the absence of any suitable computer in the west of England. The transfer of hundreds of thousands of cards to and from Imperial College, London, is the least satisfactory part of the procedure. When the large quantities of data have been dealt with, however, the distance factor will be of minor importance. As far as possible the computer programmes are written in a standard form, with a consequent saving of time and effort for the staff concerned. The IBM 7090/94 computer at Imperial College, although a very large and versatile machine, is, however, better suited to scientific calculations than to data analysis. The backing store comprises magnetic tapes only and no random access magnetic storage medium is available. The need to present and store data in serial form restricts the methods of processing which may be employed.

In spite of these difficulties a basic nucleus of experience and methods has been established at Exeter as a result of the Community Health Research Project. Using this as a foundation the research activities could be expanded to provide a most valuable tool for the management of the health services in the locality. Directions in which immediate progress might be made include:

(i) Maintenance of an integrated personal medical record for the local population by the collection and linkage of standard records from general medical practitioners, hospitals, and local authority health departments;

(ii) The implementation of screening and surveillance programmes;

(iii) The implementation and control of admission and appointments systems for general practitioners, hospitals and local authority clinics;

(iv) A comprehensive information system within the hospital and out-patient clinic in order to assist in the care and management of the patient and in the administration of hospital services;

(v) Activity planning, both in terms of current demands, and also for prediction of trends in the pattern of medical care required in the community.

Any transfer from a research to routine basis would, however, present certain fundamental problems and the methods currently in use for items such as patient identification would almost certainly require modification. Development studies are currently being undertaken with a view to setting up a service in due course. If an operation of this type is to be undertaken, a large computer with multiple access points in general practices, hospital departments, laboratories, and local authorities would be required. It would operate on a 'real time' basis and information about significant events in the care and management of the patient and other aspects of the medical services would be captured as they occurred.

Finally, it is clear that the operation of a large scale Community Research Project of this kind involves the co-operation of virtually the whole of the medical and administrative staff in the locality. The position at Exeter is a particularly happy one in this respect and it is encouraging that so many of the consultants and general practitioners have found it possible to take part and, even more, that none has 'dropped out' during the morbidity survey year.

References

1. Medical Research Council (1961). *Instructions for the Use of the Short Questionnaire on Respiratory Symptoms*, 1960 (Committee on the Aetiology of Chronic Bronchitis).
2. World Health Organisation (1955). *International Statistical Classification of Diseases, Injuries, and Causes of Death* (seventh edition).